To

with love

Doug Perry

# Quantum Healing

# Quantum Healing

Doug Perry

**To order additional copies of this book, contact:**
Xlibris Corporation
1-888-795-4274
www.Xlibris.com
Orders@Xlibris.com
66225

# CONTENTS

# Preface

Quantum healing is as easy to learn and do as breathing. To use the naturally occurring energy systems of the body is as easy to become comfortable with as the control of your breath. When we are all first born, we find it a challenge to master the filling and emptying of our lungs with air; and after the first few successful breaths, we simply continue doing the same thing for as long as we live. You did it with breathing to sustain your physical body with the oxygen that you need for metabolism and to discharge the gaseous metabolic wastes that your body creates. It was simple because your body is designed to give you control over all the muscles and tissue that need to function so that you can breathe. It is also true for all of your life force energy systems.

Learning to become familiar with, and to control, the life force energy systems of our body is as easy as breathing. To some extent, it is happening unconsciously for all of us all the time. Some people have natural strengths in some areas of their awareness, or unconscious utility, of some aspects of their life force energy systems. As such, they may be aware of what is commonly called psychic gifts, or abilities. All of us have the potential, but most of us were trained out of believing in our gifts at very early ages. In modern and postmodern society, the mainstream beliefs are taught to all children through our education system and all people through the media like TV, radio, magazines, newspapers, Internet news. In most of these teachings, people are told that physical and financial phenomena are real and psychic and/or life force energy phenomena are fantasy or suspect of being fantasy. So most people never take the time to learn about the psychic or life force energy systems of the body.

In modern times, many people are known/purported to be able to do psychic readings or see auras or perform "medical intuitive" health analysis. There are courses that teach all three of these abilities, and anyone can learn them. Gaining these abilities is simply becoming able to utilize a few of the normal abilities available to us all. Many of those who are good enough to earn their living performing these extrasensory perception skills don't have a full understanding of how they do it or of how to activate and/or utilize all their life force energy systems. Some of them have a vast understanding of what their "gifts" have taught them, and a few have an in-depth understanding of many aspects of the various energy systems that make up the human form. But most people simply go through life ignoring their psychic gifts and energetic abilities and occasionally notice them without acknowledging their worth.

Learning to utilize our energy systems first requires a familiarity with them. That is what I/we teach first in the quantum healing seminars and classes. A familiarity is different from an understanding. Coming to understand that was the turning point in my learning that occurred shortly after a great truth was imparted upon me. Dada G explained to me years ago in my yoga training that the ratio of 95 percent practical and 5 percent intellectual was the relative scale of importance of the material that I was learning with him. Becoming familiar with the application of that ratio allowed me to begin a journey of truths. It wasn't long after realizing that the practical was the best test of the intellectual that I started to realize the power of understanding that one simple truth. So I confidently write that a familiarity with your life force energy systems is infinitely more important than an understanding of your life force energy systems.

Admittedly, an understanding of our life force energy systems can lead to a familiarity of them, but not necessarily. However, a familiarity of them will inevitably, perhaps over time, lead to an understanding of them. So that is why I have designed the course using the most practical of the information and techniques from the many various trainings I have taken. Within the course, the practical is taught first. Then a succinct explanation of the theory is added to explain the physics of the energetics. The information that is necessary to achieve the results from performing the quantum healing techniques is minimal. The actual practice is easy. But actually achieving the result requires that the steps be performed at least reasonably well. That is why a familiarity with the life force energy systems of your own body is required.

In this book, I explain the theory first then explain the techniques. The reason for the divergence from the method that has proven most successful in the classroom is that this is not a classroom. It is a book. Here, both time and the use of the information is in your control, and you can't get any feedback or input about what you are doing with your energy from the teacher (in this case, a book). In the classes, the teacher is able to watch/see what you are doing with your energy and give you feedback and guidance. Also, in the class all the material and its applications are instructed in a step-by-step procedure that ensures that you are able to perform each aspect of the material correctly before learning the next part. Also, in the classroom the various debates that may occur regarding the theory can be, and often are, time consuming and disruptive for the course and progress in the class. After people have successfully performed the practice, the theory seems to easily make sense even if they have been told contradictory descriptions of the energetics from other teachings. By allowing you the information on the theory and intellectual understanding of the energy work before giving you the techniques, I hope to enable you to perform the techniques correctly to obtain a satisfactory result for you and so that you can achieve the same energetic that is taught in the classes.

The practice material in this book will first outline and then suggest detailed mental and/or energy exercises to be attempted. It will/may describe the details of the exercises in several different terminologies as I have found that many people have varying backgrounds and some have practices that may be similar in some aspects. I have witnessed that those who have done something similar consistently realize the benefits of doing these exercises as prescribed in my teachings. And I recommend that after all those who learn this system go on to learn all that they can by comparing and experimenting with it in conjunction with other things that they have learned. But in order to understand the teachings offered here, it is necessary to perform the techniques as prescribed. The success of each new exercise will be dependent on the utilization of the previous work to achieve the energetic and vibrational state to enable easy execution of each new technique.

# Acknowledgments

Thank you to the many masters and teachers and students and strangers and events that I have been fortunate to learn from. Acquiring the information that made it possible for me to understand what I needed to develop the course that this book covers took me many years. I had no idea that my life would unravel the way it has. Like a bundle of scrolls with the secrets from many sects and societies and trainings of old, all laid before me as if pieces of a puzzle with a story waiting to be told. I would not have believed life could be so wonderful. Yes, I have always seen the beauty in all things, but the unraveling of it all can be so special and joyous when we take the time to notice and live out our passions.

Each time I found a passion and followed it through, each time was a journey of learning some truth, and I grew. With another lesson, my foundation more broad, my ability to understand came sharper and more able to pierce the gray fraud. A new day, a new dawn, a new meal of some facts and with each drink of some truth, and some time to relax and digest what my life was bringing my way. It all seemed like a barrage of strange battles in an ill-conceived play. With each new challenge departed from the last, both in direction and behavior of the cast. I soon learned to move forward at whatever the cost; as the cost would grow worse, the longer I stayed stagnant and scared without taking a choice and making an action of movement or words. But action and movement gives freedom to birds and us if too be so bold as to hear our intuition and do as we are told. So now on my journey, the travels go on, so far from the start, and the end cannot come. I've let the fear go and lived in the fun so that I can now face whatever wondrous lessons will come.

Thank you for reading this passage and, thus in some small way, allowing my thoughts to influence your mind even if only for a moment so that I may have a chance to make a difference in this world and bring learning and betterment to it even if only vicariously. For that is what I can only offer and hope comes to pass. Though each life seems small in the vastness of the world, we each have the chance to make differences with each choice and action that we take. I am thankful that I have learned to do the most good I can.

# Introduction

The concept that the vibration of one thing effects the vibration of other things is what quantum healing is based on. This is called resonance and entrainment in physics. When the vibratory rate of anything is placed in proximity to anything else, the vibratory rates of the two things will naturally pull each other toward a balance.

In quantum healing, you learn how to quickly raise your resonance and sustain it at a higher level. You also learn how to direct that higher resonance anywhere you choose. By simply holding that energetic of higher vibration on or against a person, you provide them with an opportunity for their body to entrain to the higher level. When this happens, their body will spontaneously correct itself.

# Chapter One

# *Laying a Foundation of Understanding*

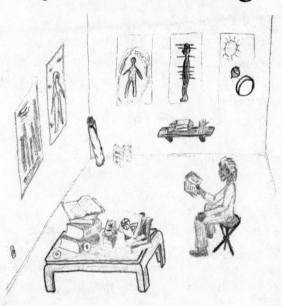

To start, I want to say that there are a lot of things to cover before we can achieve great results, and the fun stuff is a little later in the book. So let's jump ahead for a few moments and cover some important points that you won't need to know until later. Before we do that though, I want you to know that it is safe to teach the material in this book to children, as long as you understand it and can do it first yourself. Also, if you are interested in teaching this material to groups of people, it will benefit you to take the level 2 class first as lots of advanced material is covered that will make it much easier for them to follow the teachings and stay attentive during the classes. So let's get started.

A common question of many students that I have had from various Qigong or energy work modalities is, What if or how do I combine this (quantum healing) with my other energy work, and/or is it safe to do so? The answer is simply that if you do them both/all simultaneously without modifying either/any in order to do so, then they are safe to do together. And if you want to do that, then you should practice them independently alone first until you are confident and comfortable doing them independently. Then you can simultaneously perform them together until you are comfortable doing them correctly at the same time before you do it with your clients. I suggest practicing alone or with colleagues before attempting anything experimental on an unsuspecting client. But first and foremost, before trying to do something new and different, it is important to master the techniques in order to achieve the vibrational shift which occurs and get the benefits of that shift. Once you have mastered the quantum healing practice, the clarity and increased intuition will help you by making it easier to understand what you are achieving with the energy work that you are doing.

The next thing of importance to discuss here is integrity. Staying in integrity with truth and respect for all others is essential to anyone's personal growth. As you rise in vibration from this work, or other work, the way that your thoughts and actions affect your soul's journey may become more apparent to others than to you yourself. As you start to utilize your gifts and abilities more fully, the actions and thought that you choose will have greater impact on others around you and upon yourself. The karmic repercussions of manipulating others for your own gain may go unnoticed by you until a time when you are unable to undo the damage to your journey. So I suggest you take the oath I prescribe to those who take my classes. The act of taking the oath will remind you on a deep level that your actions do have impact and that it is vital to be conscious of the efforts that you take, or avoid taking, which affect others and the directions in which your actions and deeds affect them.

## Oath:

I will endeavor to live in truth and do whatever I am able to do for the benefit of others without it bringing any hardship to myself or my loved ones. I will endeavor to always consciously refrain from knowingly bringing unnecessary harm to any living thing from my actions, words, or thoughts for the rest of my life.

(Unnecessary harm—as we walk, we harm the grass and bugs, etc., that live in the grass; and all things must eat to live and all the things we eat die [at least we hope they do] when they are digested or before. So it is necessary to do some harm just to live—so it is prudent to recognize that some harm is a natural occurrence of the process of living in the physical. That being the case, it is best to forgive yourself as you cannot live a full and healthy life without actually doing some harm. But any harm that results from an act of free will that is unnecessary does have the possible effect of accumulating what is referred to as karmic debt. Harm that is unnecessary is simply any harm that is done for any purpose other than doing what is necessary to live your life in a productive and healthful manner.)

I suggest that you write out the oath and read it to yourself aloud. If it is a huge departure from the way you are living, perhaps you should read it every day for a while. If you like rituals, try it in front of a mirror, read it three times, and burn it. If you think that it is bullshit and you are going to take what you can, remember—as you sow, so shall you reap. The spiritual laws are like math. They are what they are, and the equations have variables and constants. The constants are fixed, and the variables are the result of our individual free will. If you already live in integrity, taking the oath may not seem important to you because it is the action of correct action that matters most, but taking the oath is a commitment to yourself that sets a vibration and an imprint in your unconscious that helps to allow an ease in continuing on such a path.

The wisest and most profound statement that I have yet to hear, "You don't know what you don't know," has allowed me to look beyond my beliefs, prejudices, trainings, and shortcomings to become more than I was. And it has become true that I learn as much from my students as I have from my teachers. I have learned that living in integrity with myself and others is easier than any alternative. And I always feel good about my thoughts, words, and actions. Even when I find out that I was wrong, as I know that I did what I did because I felt, believed, and thought that it was the best thing to do at the time. Following this path, I have found it true that I never regret the things that I have done; I only ever regret the things that I did not do.

There are four main reasons for doing the work in this book. The first one is that it is fun. The second is that it will enable you to grow personally faster than any other short set of exercises that you will ever find. I have seen profound changes in many of the people that have taken the sixteen-hour seminar with me and/or with the other teachers of this modality. It will truly allow you to experience life more fully and to understand your way of being and your perspectives from a broader viewpoint and a deeper level. The third is that it will allow you to help many other people with physical, emotional, and spiritual problems that they may be suffering from, as well as helping yourself with your own health. The fourth is that you will need to be able to perform the techniques in quantum healing level 1 before you can take the quantum healing level 2 class. Well, the fourth reason may not seem that important to you yet, but after working with the techniques in this book for a while, you may choose to learn even more about your life force energy systems and what they can do for you.

# Chapter Two

# *Maintaining Your Aura*

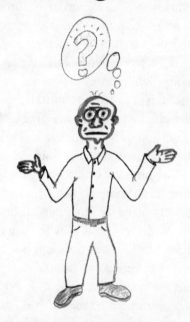

Step 1 is to bolster your energy and clean your aura. If you are fully aware of your aura, this will be easy; and if you are not sure what an aura is, this will be easy.

First, some theory. Your aura is an aspect of your being. What I mean by this is that in order to have a physical body like we inhabit here (*on the earth plane / in physical reality*), there is a complex matrix of interconnected and overlapping and intermingling energy systems that are all interacting simultaneously with each other. Each of them is functioning as designed and somewhat independent of the others, as well as having a direct and indirect influence on the functioning of the others. The aura is one of the energy systems that is actually outside of our physical body. It has no physical structure of its own except the whole physical body in its entirety. The aura has several layers. Most people, with a little training, can feel five of them and then a sixth thinner one very close to the physical body. Some people that I know who have developed their abilities can see several layers within the layers.

The colors of the human aura change according to moods, emotions, thought, health, and "stuff" in the aura and other factors. The colors can be changed as per your choice once you learn how. The color, or whatever else is, in the aura has a two-way relationship with the rest of our body. The aura has an effect of showing a reflection of what is in the body and also of projecting into the body what has entered or become present in the aura. So it is fair to say that by reading an aura, you get a true representational image of what is in the body; and conversely, what you place, or allow, in your aura has an influential effect on the physical body, emotional body, and thought forms in the body. When other life-forms, or the energetic of other life-forms, invade our aura, it starts to set a vibration that is friendly to their existence, remaining attached to or welcome in our body. This can be an early warning if we are willing to see/notice it and take action accordingly.

In my studies and experience, the way that the aura affects our beings is through its effect on our physical body. From there, what is in our aura can influence our feelings and thoughts. It has an indirect effect from there on the other aspects of our being as our physical body affects the various aspects of us. Some people have stated that the aura has direct effects on other aspects of our being, but I have not seen how, at least not yet. So I confidently conclude that the aura is our natural buffer against what all is in our energy environment in the physical world. It extends around us about three feet, or a meter. By cleaning it of the various "stuff" that gets stuck in it every day, we can usually avoid things like colds and flu. (It is safer than a vaccine and cheaper too.) We can also absorb influences from others in our aura, and cleaning this out is just as easy and important, but usually not as noticed if left to fester.

The technique that I use in quantum healing to clean the aura is an aspect of *hilot*. *Hilot* is part of what I learned when studying Philippine Shiatsu therapy. *Hilot*, as it was taught to me, is the energy work aspect of Philippine Shiatsu/acupressure massage. This technique is an aspect or part of that system. It is similar to many healing systems except for a few details. The way I utilize it may vary slightly from the way that it was meant to be practiced when it was taught to me by Datu Shishir in 1988. I have had a few students insist on doing it with their own variations; and I have tried it several, actually many, different ways. Because of the gentleness and subtle power in the way I have chosen to teach it, I will continue to teach it this way. The other variations all seemed to work but have various subtle differences in the tone of the energetic that they each produce.

This process basically takes the loving essence of the love of God, or the essence of the cosmos or heaven, along with the loving essence of the Mother Earth, or the energy of the physical existence of the planet, and merges them to fill the life-form that is like a bridge between the two very different realms of existence. Without the two energies merging in the way that they naturally do, life as we know it in physical form would not be possible. The two energies merging in the way that we do this work is in correct alignment with conscious human development to form true understanding of life as we know it in physical form and how it is possible. The thing is in this work, we will consciously allow, or control, the merging of these basic forces. In nature, they occur without any conscious effort in a much smaller and less intense flow all the time. In this work, we will increase the flow and brighten our ability to live/be alive/experience our connection with the forces of life /awaken ourselves to what we truly are. By recognizing the energetic reality that allows us the gift of life, we gain the ability to utilize some control over how much life force we have available to us.

Invite pure white light energy to come into your top from
Heaven/God/the universe/source/the cosmos
and all allow it to fill you up.

Invite clean rich pure red light energy to come from
the loving essence of the Earth
and fill you from the bottom.

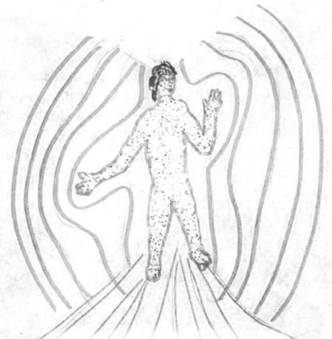

Let the white and the red light energy
merge/blend/swirl into/become one effervescent pink glow
filling your physical body.

Expand the pink glowing energy to fill your aura
displacing any inappropriate energetics.

First, allow or invite the pure white loving light from/of God/heaven/ source/the universe/above to come in through the top of your body. Allow it to fill up the entirety of your physical body. Let it fill every aspect of your physical being. Once it has filled all your organs, your bones, your muscles, your hands, feet, fingers, toes, legs, nose, arms, ears, neck, face, belly, back, and brain, make sure that it has also filled all your skin; the hair is optional.

Next, allow/invite/bring in/draw up/ask the pure loving essence of Mother Earth/the planet to enter the bottom of your body as a brilliant clean red light/ energy and guide or witness it, fill up the entirety of your physical being. Do this the same way that you did the white from above. So let it fill your arms, hands, fingers, toes, legs, feet, face, head, back and front, teeth, etc. The order/ sequence that you fill your body is not really important, but it seems logical to start where the light enters and fill to the farthest ends of your body.

Once your physical body is completely filled with both the white and red at the same time, then you are ready for the next step.

Next, set your intent that the white from above and the red from below will continue to flow into your physical body. Intend that they will both continue to flow in filling the entirety of your physical being completely full so that you have both the red and the white filled to the outermost edges of all of your skin at the same time.

Next, as the red and white continue to fill your body fully, allow the red and the white to merge together and form a beautiful effervescent pink glow. Allow/make/ask/visualize/guide the red and white to merge/mix/swirl/ transform/meld/bond into the pink effervescent glow. Allow the white and red to continue entering the top and bottom of your physical being and continue melding them into the pink effervescent glow. Allow that beautiful pink to fill your entire body/physical being so that it is packed into every aspect of your entire physicality.

Next, while you allow the white and the red to continue to flow into and fill up your body completely, and you have the white and red in your body transforming to become the effervescent pink glow, allow that pink glow to start to expand out beyond the confines of your physical being to fill up your aura. Slowly allow the pink glow to start filling out from all directions, from all aspects of your physical body at the same time. It is OK to only notice it expanding out from one area at a time at first. While you witness, or watch, or feel it expanding out beyond your skin to fill your aura, notice if it displaces any other energies or lights or spaces with a lack of light. While you allow the pure white and red to enter from the top and bottom and mix to become the pink, continue to let it fill out to completely fill your aura.

If at first when you do this exercise you don't see or feel the colors, it is OK. If at first when you do this you don't get a sense of the energies and all that you do is imagine that you are doing it, that is OK. In Yoga theology, it is taught that as thought is created, energy follows. Or energy follows thought. Your imagination is one of the most powerful tools of your mind. If you only imagine that you are doing the exercise, most people who see in energy will be able to witness that you are in fact moving the energy, transforming the energy, and changing the dynamic of your entire energy field.

After imagining that you are doing the entire exercise a few times, imagine that you could see and feel the energy and imagine what it does look and feel like. You will find that as you imagine what it does look and feel like, you will get an accurate image and perception of how it looks and feels. If you regularly utilize your imagination in this manner, it will only take a short time until you are clearly getting a true perception of what the energy looks and feels like. While some people immediately are able to see or feel or hear the energy, others have to imagine that they can and see and feel how it would look or feel or sound if they were perceiving it. Some folks "try" to see it for decades and never really get good at it. (*To try is to accept the possibility of failure—as long as you accept the possibility of failure, the messages in the unconscious mind that tell us that we can't and don't see auras or energy will prevent us from perceiving auras and energy.*) By imagining that we *do* see and *do* feel energy, we allow our unconscious mind to accept the truth that we are willing to perceive the aura and energy so it allows us to *do* so. Basically, by utilizing our imagination in this manner, we trick our unconscious mind to bypass the restrictions that have been imposed on our abilities to be aware of various aspects of the world that surrounds us.

Once the pink has completely filled the entire aura to the point of noticing, *or if imagining that you can notice when you imagine that you are noticing,* that the density of the pink is intensely packed to the extreme outer limit of your aura (your aura extends about three feet, or a meter, out from your skin in all directions from all aspects of your body), your aura is clean. That simple exercise is all that is necessary to clear and/or clean your aura. There are other methods of cleaning and/or clearing auras in other modalities, and they all work. Some require putting your hand in the aura to move and shift the energies. Some are done with the help of spirit guides. Some take a great deal of effort, and others are easy. They all seem to work.

In addition to cleaning your aura, this technique also connects you with the heaven and earth energies. In the foundations of Chinese medicine, it is sort of explained how our physical form is where heaven and earth meet.

As such, it is vital that we are in connection with both energies so that we can stay in balance/healthy. By inviting both the heaven and earth energies into our physical form at the same time and merging them, we are actually bolstering the natural processes of energetics that are required to maintain and run our bodies. So at the same time that we are cleaning any incorrect energy off our body and out of our aura, we are giving our body some of the energy which it needs to maintain itself.

Before                                          After

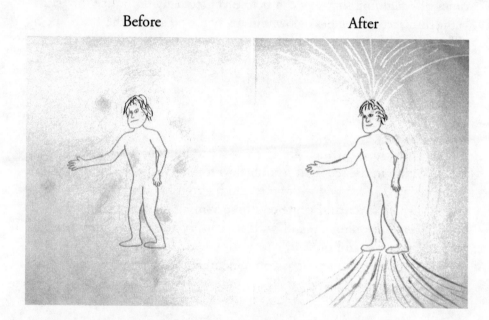

In quantum healing, it is essential that you clear your aura first before working on yourself or a client. The other energy work will work if you don't, but if you don't clean your own energy before you start to do the other aspects of the quantum healing techniques, the "stuff" that may be attached to you can facilitate you being easily distracted during the session, and that can lead to a lesser result than is normal. To achieve the energetic that allows the "quantum healing" to take place requires a certain amount of participation and concentration from the practitioner. Often the "stuff" that is sometimes stuck on us or in our auras can influence our minds to wander and sometimes even fixate on things that truly are not of real interest to who we really are. I wouldn't expect that anyone constantly runs the heaven and earth energy to fill their body and auras with that effervescent pink glow. But it does feel good if you do. I do ask that you always do it before doing a healing on another or yourself and during the treatment/session if you are willing. If you do it after a session or each session, it will ensure that nothing that comes off a client during a session can become attached to you.

If the first few times you do this you are so busy doing the technique that you don't, or hardly do, notice that the pink is moving "stuff" out of your aura, that is normal. Once you become familiar with the process and comfortable doing the techniques, you will start to easily perceive the "stuff" that gets displaced if it is in your aura. Sometimes it takes several times of imagining that you can before you actually do notice the "stuff" being displaced by the pink glow. But many people notice the "stuff" being cleared off the first, second, third, or fourth time that they do the technique. Of course, if they do it a couple of times in a row, there is nothing to notice as their energy and aura are both pretty clean.

So a recap:

1. Bring in the white light from above to fill your body completely.
2. Bring in the red light from bellow to fill your body completely.
3. Have the red and white mix and fill your body with pink.
4. Have the red and white continue coming in and mixing.
5. Have the pink expand with its density to displace any incorrect energetics and fill your entire aura.
6. Continue and repeat as you remember to.
7. Imagine that you do it all the time without any effort.

# Chapter Three

# *The Basic Energetic*

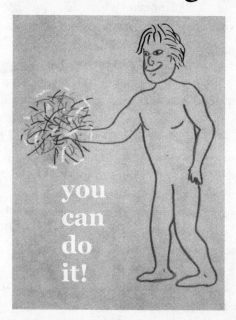

you
can
do
it!

The next aspect of achieving a heightened vibrational state via the quantum healing method is to utilize an active body awareness technique. This technique has similarities to practice and exercises in many various yoga, Qigong, biofeedback, and new age teachings. The main thing that is different here is the specific way that the awareness is focused and repeated. Or one may say that the difference is the way that the awareness is repeatedly focused. The procedure of repetition, intensity, and sequence of the awareness is how the result is achieved. Once you learn how to do this, it is very easy and almost does itself for you.

Anytime that you become aware of an aspect of your body, it is correct to say that you have brought it into your awareness. Simply semantics, yes? Well, I want to talk about the importance of that so that it will make more sense later. To be aware or to think about or feel or experience an aspect of ourselves is to fix an aspect of our mind's attention upon it. Our attention is an energetic. Just like ideas are energetics and thoughts are energetics. Once you train yourself to see in energy, you may start to see the energetics of ideas pass from one person to another when they are having conversations. Anyway, when you bring your attention onto another energetic, it can sometimes have an effect on that other energetic just by it (your attention) being present.

For example, when you pay attention to a pet or child, they often notice even if you don't touch them or make any noise. If you bless your food or "put love into it while you are cooking," it makes it taste better, at least some say so. If you talk to your plants, they grow better, but they don't have ears, do they? These are examples of how your attention affects other energetics. Now modern physics succinctly states that all matter is made up of energy, so all matter is actually energy holding a solid form. That ability of that energy to congeal into a solid state and remain stable in that solid state requires the energetic pattern of a specific type to be present and acting specifically on that energy so that it does not transform into anything else. Do you see what I mean? Any way, all things are made of energy, and sometimes when two energetics interact, a third is created.

When I was in about grade 2, we learned to make a magnet by stroking one nail over another. To make a comparison, what we were doing was dragging or moving one energetic (a nail) across the other energetic (the other nail) to make a third energetic—the third energetic being the magnetic field. The third energetic was very different from the first two as it was not a physical structure. Although the magnetic field has no actual physical structure, it is associated with the physically solid structure of the one nail. When we drag our attention across our physical body, we get a similar effect. Not the same, but similar. The one energetic—our attention—is dragged or pushed against the second energetic (our physical body), and an energy field is created. Not a magnetic field but an energy field that is of the vibration of the correctness of design of our living body and its life force.

I have seen variations of this technique used in several energy healing systems. The simplest variation is a light soft vigorous rubbing or brushing of a sore area. This is common to several massage traditions as a minor aspect of the therapy. I met a woman who explained that in her Qigong training they learned a specific technique to slowly move the energy through their body and to their hands to create a great heat that produced a healing effect for most conditions. In some martial arts systems healing techniques are taught that are somewhat similar in practice and effect. Like the healing shown in the movie *The Karate Kid* the master moves energy down his arms to his hands while making a dramatic clap of his hands and then rubs them together before placing them on his injured student, or client. I had seen and tried some variations of these healing techniques before I saw that film and had been able to achieve results from all of them.

I also trained in and taught Quantum-Touch where they do something very similar to what is taught here. While I was a teacher, the Quantum-Touch administration quite adamantly stated that what I was doing was not their system, and they discontinued my teaching status. Apparently, I had misunderstood some of the details of their technique when I took the classes from their founder. It seemed that the method that they had learned from Bob Rasmussen was taught in a less than concise manner, to me anyway. All the students that I taught the variation to had gotten good results in the classes, and I heard some stories from a few of them later about astounding results that they achieved with their clients using the methods that I had taught. To make a long story short—after teaching it for a year, I was told that I was doing it wrong, so I did some experimentation with variations of the techniques and found that it was different and that it worked very well. At that time, I was surprised and saddened to be forbidden to teach for them. However, this allowed me to add a lot of new information and advanced teachings to the classes. I called my classes quantum healing. I have taught this, my method, for several years now and have been seeing consistent good results without any resulting problems or side effects for the clients or practitioners.

Basically the "waves of awareness" aspect of quantum healing is very easy and straightforward. You simply feel your body or experience how every aspect of your physical body feels as fully as you can while you inhale. The sequence of feeling the body is what is important. You feel how your body feels from your feet to the crown of your head and then to your hands while you inhale. So basically, you take your attention to explore the experience of how each part of your body feels, exploring the various sensations that every tissue and every type of cell in your entire body feels, just a few at a time. Well, that is the theory. In actual practice, the sections of your body may *kind of seem that they are* a sequence rather than a large group of separate parts.

Starting at your feet, you feel how your toes feel (with your mind, not your hand). Bring your attention to experience your toes, toenails, webs between your toes, bones of your toes, muscles, tendons, and skin of your toes, then your soles of your feet. At the soles of your feet, you notice how your skin feels, how the joints between the bones of the foot feels, the instep and the outside of the foot, the top of the foot, the ankle, etc. Follow the process all the way up through the internal organs to the crown of the head, and then without stopping, you continue feeling each aspect down the sides of the head and down the arms to the hands.

After explaining the technique, I will write a step-by-step procedure that can be followed for practicing the various techniques in all their separate parts and how to practice them together all at once. As you learn to do each aspect of this technique and practice it a couple of times, you will become able to incorporate the next aspect of the system easily. If you read through it all first, it may seem like a lot of things to be doing all at once, and you will be correct. We are all doing a lot of things all at once all the time anyway. We are controlling our breath, digesting whatever we ate, storing calories as fat, retrieving minerals from our bones, placing other minerals in our bones, regulating our heartbeats and vein elasticity to circulate our blood, controlling our anal and bladder sphincters, controlling our eyelids and our irises to determine the amount of light entering our eyes, controlling the muscles that adjust our lens so that our eyes are able to collect a clear image to send the signals to the optical aspect of our brain where it is interpreted. We are feeling the pressure of the many constant pulses on our eardrums and interpreting those patterns into sounds, we are accepting particles from the air into membranes in our nostrils and calculating their origins in our olfactory nerves to give us the sense of smell, and we are holding our body in some sort of position (correct or slouching) with some of the muscles that we seldom consciously control, we are feeling every aspect of our body and returning commands for our tissue to perform functions, and we are most likely daydreaming just a little bit—at least between our thoughts.

At first, each action of our life force energy systems that we bring into our consciousness/conscious control may seem a little difficult. The second time that we bring an action or activity of our life force energy systems into our conscious control may seem easy, but we might not notice much else that is happening. By the third time we do a new thing in energy work with our own life force energy systems, it usually seems like it is an easy and comfortable activity, and we can be fully aware of all that is occurring around us. Well, at least as fully as before we learn to handle the new activity of our life force energy systems. So in this manner, I will ask you to practice the new techniques; do each new activity three times then move on to the next.

In the classes, we only practice each new technique twice, but we have a master of this system observing and assisting with each step and overlooking the vibe of the room, etc., to assure easy and correct learning. If you are learning this alone from this text, you will benefit from the extra few minutes of practice, and it will help give you some of the understanding that you may receive from listening to feedback and directions from all the people who would be present in a class.

After bringing your attention and/or awareness through your body from your feet to your crown on top of your head to your hands as you inhale, you exhale, noticing how your hands and the area around them feels. You do that for several breaths in a row without holding your breath in or out for any pause time between. So you do that as you take slow, easy, deep breaths inhaling through the mouth. Did I mention inhaling through the mouth? I am now. I accept that it may be different for some, but do it inhaling through the mouth, and after you become comfortable with this method, see if you notice a difference inhaling through the nose only.

To do this technique correctly, you must only feel, or notice, how your body actually feels in a sequence starting from the feet to the head then to the hands as you inhale through your mouth. The more fully you feel your physicality, the better you are doing this technique. The sequence is important as it determines where the energetic will be created. For variations on this, check appendix 2.

The wave of awareness is simply bringing your attention to sense how your body feels following a sequence, starting from the feet and ending in the hands as follows; or in a similar manner. Big toes, toes, bottom of feet, insteps, top of feet, bones and muscles in feet, skin of feet, front of ankles, out side of ankles, Achilles' tendon, inside of ankles the skin, the bones, the front of the shin, bones, out side of the shins, calves of the legs, inside of the calves and shins, the skin, the knee caps, skin of the knees, back of the knee, knee joints, bottom of the thigh, outsides of the thighs, back of the legs, muscles, bones, skin, the inside of the thighs, bottom of the torso, anus and the genitals, the hips the tendons, tissue around the hips, the buttocks, sacrum, large intestine, bladder, pelvic bone, tummy skin and muscles on the sides of the belly, the floating ribs, lower back spine, the kidneys and intestines, spleen and liver, the abdominal muscles, ribs, middle back, vertebra of the middle back, heart, stomach, pancreas and gallbladder, the sternum, the chest or breasts, and skin, underarms, scapula and upper back, the vertebra, lungs, bronchia, esophagus, throat, the back of the mouth the jaw, tongue, nose face, brain, sinuses, skull and eyes, forehead, top of the head, scalp, ears, sides of the neck, shoulders, biceps, inside of the arms, the skin the bone the triceps, the elbows, the creases of the elbows, funny bone, for-arm, the muscles and tendons, bones, skin, the wrists, the back of the hands, palms the muscles and the tendons, bones and skin, the fingers and thumbs.

*Feel how your body feels (inside) from your feet, ankles, legs, torso, neck, head, neck, shoulders, arms, hands. Feel each part of your body in sequence from the feet to the head to the hands. Then notice how your hands feel.*

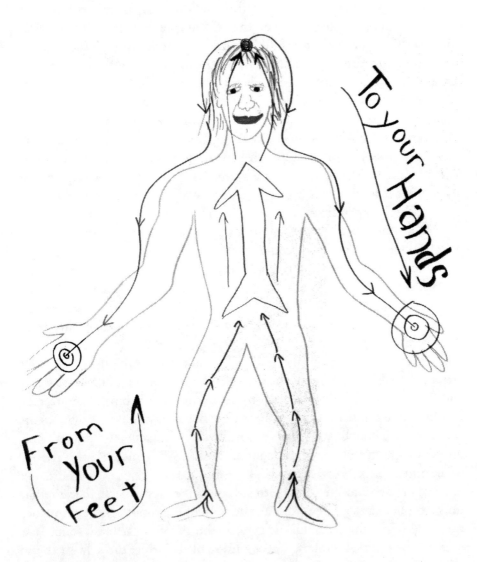

The reason that I ask you to do this inhaling through the mouth is that most of the people who do this, about 90 percent, clearly notice and admit that they notice a greater energy intensity in the end result if they do it inhaling through the mouth rather than through the nose. I know that with several specific practices that the nose is used to draw air in using specific practices and procedures to achieve specific results, and I know how well it actually works. This is different. This actually works better through the mouth. Of the 10 percent that don't admit that the breathing through the mouth seems to work better for this technique, most of them were uncertain that there was a difference that they could notice and that they stated that they "could not feel the difference." And the rest—only a few—seemed to either have had a greater effect or experienced a greater effect or believed that they were having a greater effect by not breathing through the mouth. So after you become comfortable and familiar with doing this simple technique while inhaling through the mouth only, try it in other ways and see what your experience is.

After doing the waves of awareness from the feet to the head to the hands during your inhale through the mouth for about twelve to twenty breaths, three times, you will be ready for the next step. By the third time, you may have a good sense of the energetic that you are creating around your hands. On the second and third round of this exercise, you should simply focus your attention to feel or notice or sense the way that the energy/energetic feels or looks around your hands (if you are psychically sighted [appendix 3]). By the third attempt, you may be getting a sensation that you could describe. If not, then as you are doing the third round of this exercise, imagine that you can feel or sense the energetic around your hands that you are creating with this technique and ask yourself something like "What does this energetic feel or look like around my hands?" and imagine that you can see or feel it as your unconscious mind searches for the answer for you.

There is another method of coming to recognize what the energy that is starting to accumulate around your hands feels like. By continuing the technique without putting any expectation that there may be an effect or sensation to feel or even notice and starting to let your mind wander—while you continue the technique—you will likely eventually reach a state of boredom with the mind wandering, and a Zen or Zen-like state will eventually be reached. If you continue to practice the technique correctly through that process—and after—you may eventually notice the sensation around your hands. This process is not going to work every time, and it can take a long time to go through this process. But the technique does work, and others can see and feel the energetics that you will be creating around your hands, so they are there. That is why I like to use the imagine method—it is quick and almost always effective the first time.

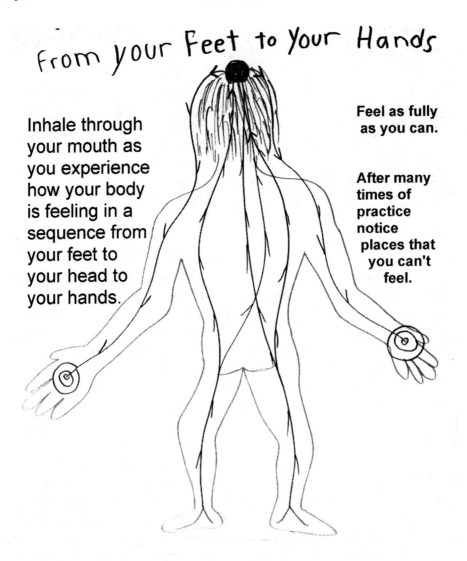

# From your Feet to your Hands

**Inhale through your mouth as you experience how your body is feeling in a sequence from your feet to your head to your hands.**

**Feel as fully as you can.**

**After many times of practice notice places that you can't feel.**

On the third time of doing this exercise, I suggest that you start to notice areas of your body that are more difficult to feel as your waves of awareness flow past them. If you find areas that you can't really feel or don't feel very fully or don't seem to have any feeling as your waves of awareness move over/through them, notice where those places are. The places that you are less able to feel are places where you have blocks of some kind. Those places are where you may want to do some work on yourself later. As you bring your conscious awareness to these areas by doing the waves of awareness in this healing modality, you are actually opening those areas ever so slightly to release those blocks. Sometimes, not often but sometimes, just doing the waves of awareness during this work can be enough to release old blocks and healing can occur.

Next, you can start to focus on having the energetics that you feel around your hands spin as spheres around your hands while you are exhaling from each breath. If you are one of the one in a hundred or so that can't feel or sense a damned thing but is willing to continue on faith alone, that is OK. Just start, or keep, imagining that you do feel, sense, see, know, hear, or in any other way are aware of the energetics that you are dealing with. The ability to have full awareness in energy is in every one of us, and we are all able to achieve these abilities. It is simply a matter of overcoming the unconscious programming that has our mind not recognizing that these energetics are within the scope of our senses.

I was one who had to go on faith for several months of Qigong practice before I could feel anything at all in energy. I had seen the result of some very good practitioners/masters and believed that they were really doing something. I had no idea what they were doing; but I saw, and felt, the results, so I was given the reason to have faith. I saw the results but did not feel the energy for many weeks and didn't start to see it for more than a year. I had my faith and my youthful exuberance, so I practiced diligently until I did sense the energy.

Most of my students feel or see the energy before the level 1 classes are over, but some have a hard time believing/admitting to themselves that they did. In giving feedback, many students can describe the color and/or shape of energy and/or how it feels to them. But when asked directly "Can you see or feel the energy?" some of the same students answered no. In my studies of NLP and hypnotherapy, I came to understand that this is simply an effect of the unconscious mind holding on to a lot of information that contradicts the new experience. In some instances when I reminded them of their description of the energy after they stated that they were unable to sense it, they got very confused looks on their faces. A couple of students went on to restate their description of the energy that they sensed and then restated that they could not see or feel energy and then looked quite perplexed. The unconscious mind never distinguishes truth from fantasy; it simply stores data into and retrieves information from the complete log of all that we have been exposed to. If we have been taught that we don't see or feel energy, that is what our unconscious mind will tell us if we put the question to it. But if we are seeing it, or feeling it, we can have clarity on what we are feeling or seeing and can describe those feelings and images. It is similar to how we can love and hate something or someone at the same time. It defies logic, so eventually we choose one or the other, and that choice usually determines what our unconscious mind will tell us the next time it is asked.

Before I learned how to sense energy or energetics, I was doing a basic chi-absorbing exercise that I was directed to do for twenty minutes a day. One night, I did it for about forty-five minutes before stopping. After I stopped doing the Qigong and started to walk around, I realized that I was feeling intoxicated. It kind of felt like being drunk but without the heavy feeling from alcohol. It only lasted about fifteen minutes, but I felt great afterward and all of the next day. After that, I started to feel the subtle sensations of the energy building up in parts of my body and around my body each time I did that exercise. It took some concentration to discern the slight variation in the way that I was feeling to determine that I was noticing "the energy" at first. But once I came to recognize what it was that I was feeling and how it felt, I was able to open my mind to accept that new aspect of my environment and explore it at will.

The next aspect of the quantum healing technique is to take control of the energetic around your hands and move it. We will be spinning those energy fields as balls around our hands. There are three main purposes for this. First, it makes the energy fields more dynamic so they sustain longer and are more noticeable. Second, it allows the practitioner an opportunity to expand their awareness to include the energy that they have created around their hands and to work with this new awareness to expand their ability to sense energy and become aware of the subtle differences that can be presented in various energetics. Third, the sustained energy balls create a high-vibration energy barrier between the practitioner and the incorrect energetics leaving the clients. This third purpose is the one that becomes important when you are treating clients with serious health issues. Because the spinning, more dynamic energy balls sustain longer, they provide the practitioner with a protective energy barrier for a short time after the session ends, which allows the practitioner to deal with/clean up the energy in the room after each session.

For the most part any negative, incorrect, or pathological energetics that are removed or disintegrated or transformed during a session of quantum healing are rendered harmless and cannot affect anyone; but this is not always the case. So this spinning is a useful aspect of the practice.

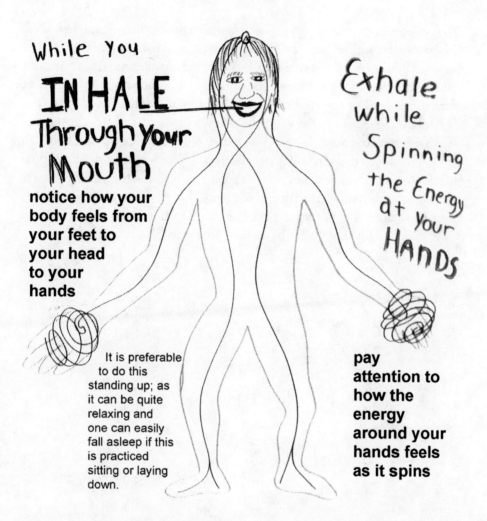

While You

# IN HALE
## Through your
## Mouth

**notice how your
body feels from
your feet to
your head
to your
hands**

*Exhale
while
Spinning
the Energy
at Your*
## HANDS

It is preferable
to do this
standing up; as
it can be quite
relaxing and
one can easily
fall asleep if this
is practiced
sitting or laying
down.

**pay
attention to
how the
energy
around your
hands feels
as it spins**

So you will continue to experience your whole body with your attention from your feet to your head to your hands as you inhale through your mouth, and then during the exhale of each breath, you will imagine/visualize/tell/make/ask/have the energy balls that you've formed around your hands spin in any direction. The direction that you have them spin in is up to you, and there is no best direction. Sometimes the balls will have a direction that they start spinning that is prior to you choosing a direction. That's OK. I have seen that the direction of the balls spin is totally under your control if you are willing to take that control (and if you are not willing to take control, perhaps you should take a look at the areas of your life where you are not willing to take control and come to understand why).

Did you know that everything in nature spirals when it travels? Well, objects, fluids, and air anyway. Birds, animals, and fish may not spiral, but the wind and the water in rivers and streams do. As does the blood in your veins. The spiraling movement has a result of somehow allowing more efficient movement through matter and energy too. That is why they put feathers on the ends of arrows so that they will spiral and thus go farther and straighter. And why do they put the laces on the side of a football? To grip it in order to make it spiral when thrown. When energy spirals, it goes farther and straighter too. That is why we are now going to spiral our waves of awareness from our feet to our heads to our hands. When you get used to spiraling the waves, you may experience a shift in the intensity and volume of the energy balls that you spin around your hands as you exhale.

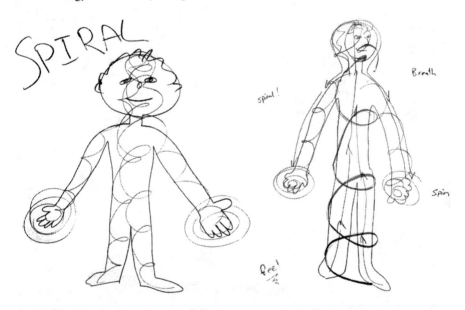

There are two ways to spiral the waves of awareness. One is to feel how your body feels from your feet to your head to your hands in a spiraling manner. Meaning that you take your attention through your body, feel the sensations that are there, following a spiraled process of feeling one part of yourself and then the next. The other way is to imagine that there is a large coil, or spiral shape, that starts at your feet and reaches to your head and then changes direction and goes to your hands. Then imagine or visualize that when you feel your body starting at your feet that your awareness goes past the spiral and follows the shape of it as it strobes from your feet to your head to your hands. Both of these methods work, and you can use them both at the same time if you like.

**As you inhale through your mouth feel how your body feels in a spiraling manner from your feet to your head and then to your hands. Bring your awareness, like a wave that is spiraling through you, from your feet to your head and then to your hands as you inhale through your mouth. As you exhale spin the energy balls around your hands; and notice how your hands feel, and how the energy around them feels.**

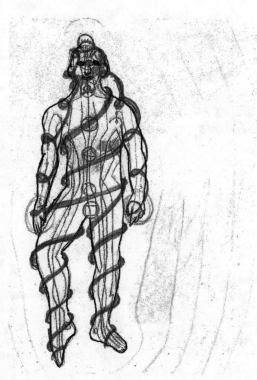

As you are spiraling your waves of awareness, bringing your waves of awareness over the internal imagined or visualized spiral or coil the dynamic of the energetic that it creates is increased. The first few times you do this technique, it may seem like a lot to do, but most people are able to perform the spiraling very well and comfortably by the third, fourth, or fifth time. If you don't notice the shifting of the energetic at first, give it a few rounds so that you become more comfortable with the technique. Then do it a few breaths without the spirals and then a few breaths with the spirals. This will help you to notice the difference.

You will most likely notice the difference. About 90 percent of the people in the classes do notice the difference by the third time they spiral their waves of awareness. Some people find it much easier to spiral their waves of awareness than to do the waves without the spiral. A few people have some difficulty achieving a good spiraling technique. Once you are comfortable with the spiral technique, it becomes easier, and you are soon able to do it very quickly. Almost all students have all been comfortable doing the spiral through most of the rest of the seminar. By the end of the sixteen-hour course, most students are doing the spiral technique all the time without seeming to have to put out any effort at all. The result is denser and more radiant energy balls that you are able to spin around your hands.

Now that you are comfortable with the spiraling of your waves of awareness as you inhale through your mouth, and the spinning of the balls around your hands while you exhale, you are ready for the next step. Now you are going to do more than one wave of awareness with each inhale through the mouth. The more the merrier, so let's get to it.

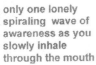
only one lonely spiraling wave of awareness as you slowly inhale through the mouth

two spiraling waves on the inhale through the mouth

four spiraling waves on the inhale through the mouth

six spiraling waves on the inhale through the mouth

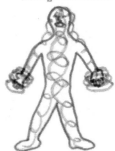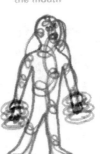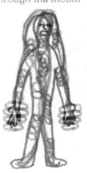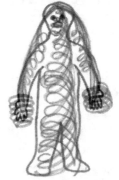

exhale slowly enough to focus on spinning the balls of energetic for four times as long as you inhaled while you were bringing the wave of awareness to your hands

spinning the balls three times as long as you inhaled

Spinning/exhale only as long as it took to feel the four waves on the inhale

spin the balls around your hands just as long as it took for you to bring all six waves of awareness from your feet to your head to your hands while you were inhaling through your mouth

In the class, we do exercises with one wave on the inhale and a much-slower, longer exhale with copious focus on the spinning of the balls in the hands on the exhale. Two waves on the inhale and then a much slower exhale. We do each of these "waves with breath" patterns several times so that it becomes comfortable before we attempt the next. The next takes a little more concentration at first, but everyone to date has quickly mastered it in the classes. Well, a few people claimed that it was difficult when they first tried; they seemed to have it down very well before the end of that class. Four waves of awareness on the inhale and the same amount of time on the exhale is the next pattern. And six waves on the inhale and the same amount of time on the exhale is the last pattern that we practice in the classes. After each student becomes comfortable with the various breath/wave patterns, I suggest to them that they can do more as per their personal capability.

The various breath patterns have a variety of purposes. One is to incrementally allow each student to become comfortable with a higher number of waves of awareness per breath. Another is to build a keener awareness of one's breathing and bring the students' breathing habits into their consciousness. Another is to demonstrate the different levels of intensity of the energetic and vibrational state that is achieved via the techniques.

Breathing is so important that every sport, art, and spiritual practice has some training in how to breathe or how to use breath to achieve some effect. Medical science has determined that without breath, you will die in three minutes. In Taoist and Chinese medicine, it is understood that we gather life force energy when we breathe. When they talk about absorbing life force energy, they are not talking about the oxygen that we take from the air; they are talking about chi (qi, chee, or ki [it is the same thing pronounced differently from various parts of China and Japan, etc.]).

In Taoist and Chinese/Oriental medicine, it is explained that our body gets life force energy from three places. I mention this here because they are not talking about oxygen from the air but life force energy. The first place we get life force energy is from our parents when we are conceived. There is an equation of the energetic of the available life force from the mother and the father and the place of conception at the time of conception. So the relative strengths of the three energies determine the amount of life essence or prenatal chi that is created. If the energy of all three is, or was, strong, then there will be more prenatal chi and thus a stronger constitution for the child.

In Taoist and Chinese medicine, the other two places that we naturally get chi is from our eating of food and our breathing. When we eat, it is the responsibility of the *pi* (spleen and pancreas) *qi* to energetically control digestion and derive the *gu qi* (life force energy from our food). The lungs have the task of absorbing the "gathering qi" (life force energy from the air). The lungs and the *pi*/spleen send the chi that they have collected down to the kidney where it is mixed with a minute amount of prenatal essence to produce the "upright qi." The upright qi is the chi that runs though our acupuncture meridians to energetically nourish our bodies' tissue so that it can function. In Chinese medicine, all symptoms of what we commonly call aging are treated by reactivating and/or bolstering the volume of life essence / prenatal chi.

There is a direct correlation to the abundance of prenatal chi and our vitality. It is not a simple relationship, but it is like a math equation. When there is not enough *gu qi* or gathering qi available in the equation, the prenatal chi is burned faster to make up the difference. So if you are not breathing well, you are shortening your life. It is also true that if you are not eating well, you are shortening your life, but that is not part of this course. So if you do the breathing exercises and breathe a little more fully once in a while, you will be able to enjoy life more fully longer. So here my being long-winded is in fact benefiting both of us, me by my long-windedness and you by bringing the importance of your breathing correctly to your attention again.

Also, it is true that as you collect more gathering chi, your personal energy fields become slightly more solid and are able to protect you from outside energetics like those of nature, like the wind and cold and damp. It is also true that breathing well supplies you with more oxygen and clears more metabolic waste from your blood. So even if you deny the chi information, the breathing is still a real factor for your health. In the quantum healing technique, either Taoist or Buddhist or Yoga breaths are OK. The important aspect of the breath in quantum healing is to take full deep breaths and gauge them so that you can perform several to many waves of awareness during each inhale through your mouth. And then have time to spin the energy balls around your hands on the exhales.

Remember that the more intense you are feeling the sensations that are there in your tissue as you do the waves of awareness, the greater the intensity/density of the energetic that you are creating around your hands. This is a factor that may explain, in part, why some people don't notice an increase in the energetic around their hands the first few times that they try the multiple-wave technique. As you increase the speed of the waves to perform several of them in each breath, it is easy to not notice aspects of your body when you are bringing your awareness past them. As you become comfortable with the multiple waves, and the speed that you choose to perform them at, you can easily increase the intensity of your awareness throughout the waves. It may be a challenge at first to feel your body fully as you strobe your awareness along the entire length of your body many times per breath, but after a few moments of practice, it will get much easier.

Once you become familiar with the multiple-wave technique, then you can utilize the information that you gain by noticing that some of your body is not as easy to feel as others. If a section or aspect of your body eludes awareness, or is not easily felt, that is an indication that there is likely some kind of blockage there. It could be from physical trauma, or from emotional trauma, or from external energetics getting lodged in your tissue or energetic space, or from false/incorrect thought forms holding detrimental energy patterns within your being. Whenever you notice an aspect of your body which is not easily experienced during the waves of awareness, it is information for you as to what you can work on to help your own health whenever you make the time to do so. Simply use the self-healing techniques that are in a later chapter of this book on these areas to clear the blocks when it is convenient for you to do so.

Once you are comfortable with all the techniques in this course, you can treat yourself at the same time that you work on clients, but you may find that your results are better if you focus your efforts on one person at a time. Not always, but usually. However, you can treat as many beings at a time as your skill allows.

So far, we have learned to clean our auras, create energy balls that have a healing effect, increase those energy balls' dynamic by spinning them, increase the intensity of those energy balls by spiraling our waves of awareness, and increase the density of the energetic in those energy balls by running multiple waves of awareness to them with each breath. Next, we will learn how to drastically raise our own energy vibration so that the balls we are creating will be resonating at a higher vibration because they are created from energetics of a higher vibration. Actually, you have already been doing this, as when you bring in the white and red light, it raises your vibration. It also rises a little when you merge the red and white to make pink. Your vibration rises a little when you do a wave of awareness also, but what is covered next will raise your vibration significantly higher, and each new stage of the next work raises it higher again.

To recap before we move on to the next section, so far we have cleared our energy and increased our energy with the white, red, and pink. We have learned what a wave of awareness is and how to do them. We have learned to spiral our waves of awareness and to do several waves per breath. We have learned to spin the energy balls that the waves create around our hands, and we have learned to notice how the energy balls feel. Well, at least it has been described in words and pictures, and the process of achieving the results has been outlined in detail. I hope that you have learned it; if not, practice a little more now or after you do the next sections.

Many people in the classes seem to give feedback after each new exercise which indicates that they are doing the techniques correctly and getting the correct results, yet they state that they don't think that they are doing it right. If you feel that way—that you are not sure that you are doing it right—and you have followed the instructions, then check the techniques again to be sure you are doing them the way they are stated in the book. If you are doing the quantum healing techniques as stated in the book, you are doing it right. It is as easy to do as you want it to be. People often doubt they are doing it at first, but they are doing it very well. You may be one of them. Trust yourself and practice a little. After you do the next section, it will be easier to notice the energy or the sensation of it. If you don't feel the energy, that is OK. I didn't at first either, and now many people who thought that it was bullshit have thanked me for teaching them and helping them with their health.

# Chapter Four

# *Chakras*

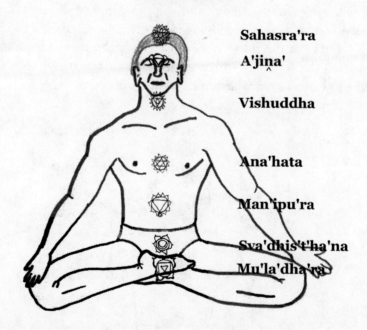

**Sahasra'ra**

**A'jina'**

**Vishuddha**

**Ana'hata**

**Man'ipu'ra**

**Sva'dhis't'ha'na**
**Mu'la'dha'ra**

Many people know about the seven internal chakras, so we will start there. The first chakra is at the perineum, at the bottom of the torso between the anus and the genitals. The second is about at the level of the pubic bone, in the center between the front and back of the body. The third is at the top of or slightly above the navel, in the center between the front and back of the body. The fourth chakra is at the level of the heart, or at the level of the nipples, in the middle of the chest, in the center between the front and back of the body. The fifth is in the center of the throat. The sixth is at about the level of the eyes or eyebrows in the center of the head. The seventh is at the top of the head. The first and seventh chakras are partially extended outside of the physical body.

The chakras are energy events that are constantly occurring. They are very dynamic in their capacities and malleable in their location and form. The chakras have no physical structure. The seven internal chakras are directly related to the function of our endocrine system. If the chakras are in balance, they induce their associated endocrine gland to function and produce the correct excretions of hormones. If the chakras are not in balance, the endocrine system is easily brought out of balance by events occurring in, and to, the physical body. As the secretions of the endocrine glands have a major influence on the functioning of most of our body's tissue, it may be wise to develop a conscious relationship with your chakras. That is what is taught in quantum healing.

The following chart is taken from yogi teachings of the chakras that I was blessed to receive while studying with Dada Sugutananda in Jamaica in 1986/7. Some of the information that I give about the chakras in the classes is from the teachings of the guru of Ananda Marga who is said to have come to earth to reestablish the teachings of Shiva.

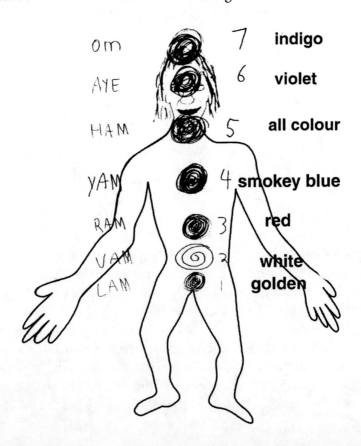

Anyway, all the information and practices that I learned from the monks have passed the test of practical application, so I utilize it. Some of the information that I convey in the classes are from various other sources and modalities that teach healings and/or practices utilizing the chakras. Some of the information that I teach in the quantum healing classes is from my own experiential learning about the chakras and has been confirmed by my students and colleagues.

Here is another chart of the chakra colors. The colors of the chakras in this chart are the ones more commonly found in popular books that teach about the chakras.

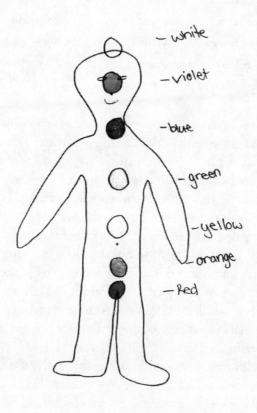

**Let's compare these charts. There are other books too with other variations of colors.**

| Chakra | Names | Color of common charts | Color of yogi charts | Sounds |
|--------|-------|------------------------|----------------------|--------|
| seventh | Sahasra'ra | white | indigo | om |
| sixth | A'jina' | violet | violet | aye |
| fifth | Vishuddha | blue | all colors | ham |
| fourth | Ana'hata | green | smoky blue | yam |
| third | Man'ipu'ra | yellow | wood-flame red | ram |
| second | Sva'dhis't'ha'na | orange | milky white | vam |
| first | Mu'la'dhu'ra | red | golden yellow | lam |

The names of the chakras are from Sanskrit as are the sounds to activate them. Sanskrit is said to be the original language spoken on earth by people. I don't know if that can be proven or disproven. Sanskrit is made up of fifty-three base sounds, and the combination of those sounds is made to make up the words so that they resonate their meaning. This is to say that when you correctly say a word in Sanskrit, the meaning or concept or intent of that word is carried as a resonance tone of accurate vibration. Or to put it another way, if you say a word in Sanskrit, the meaning of that word is broadcast through sound and thought in the energetic of the meaning of the word. That is why when you tone these sounds to activate the chakras and you hit the correct sound/tone, you can feel the resonance in the chakras.

Notice the variation in the two columns of colors in the chart. The first is the commonly publicized version of the chakra colors. There are some slight variations of it with sixth being indigo or purple or the seventh being white, purple, violet, or indigo. But the most common chakra color charts here in the West have the lower five chakras colored following the light spectrum or rainbow pattern. The Yogis had, and have, a different set of colors that they work with. As you can imagine, I have been criticized for mentioning the different colors in the chakras. I have studied and experimented to see what the difference is and have come to understand that the color of our chakras has an effect on and reflects our perspectives.

Several of my friends/colleagues who are very sighted and see the chakra colors readily have stated that the chakra colors on people change all the time. All these people have said that they seldom talk about chakra colors because those who believe but don't see like to argue about it. These arguments can easily turn personal as one party is stating what they personally experience and the other is stating what they have been taught, have worked with, and do believe to be true. So in an argument, they are both correct. So in quantum healing, you learn how to experience what color is in your chakras and how it affects the energy balls that you are creating and to put the various colors into your chakras and see if you can discern a difference in your energetics.

If you have taken some kind of training that places the chakras slightly differently, please be patient. Over the years, I have heard many different descriptions of where the chakras are and their shapes and what they do and how they work, etc. Many of the trainings were mostly intellectual in nature, and some had some practical work associated with the information, and other trainings were practically based. For years, I was wondering which system was correct. Then I learned how to develop a relationship with my chakras and become aware of what was true and what was just some slight misunderstandings.

Because our chakras have an effect on our secretions of hormones, they have a grand effect on our physical well-being; and through how that affects the energy balances in our organs, they have a very real effect on our emotions. And because they also host our perceptions, they have a secondary indirect effect on how we feel. They also have an effect on how we interact with our surroundings. How conscious we are in our relating with our chakras determines our conscious control on all these areas.

To do the exercises to build a relationship with our chakras, it is best if you are standing. The reason is that if you are sitting or lying down, especially in a very comfortable position, you will likely gently float off into a nice, peaceful sleep. The reason for this is that as you raise your vibration, your brain wave patterns change. As the frequency of your brain waves respond to the raised vibrational state that is induced by the chakra work, they will become similar in amplitude to that of sleep, and your unconscious mind will react by allowing you to fall asleep very easily. If you are standing, your unconscious mind will also have the information that you are always awake when you are standing, so it will make it easier to stay alert while you become comfortable at the new higher vibrational state. That is why in the monasteries of old, one monk would walk between the rows of those doing sitting meditations and nudge, tap, or hit those who had fallen asleep. It wasn't a punishment, only a way of training them to remain conscious.

# Five External Chakras

## ~ Soul Chakras ~

## Eighth, Ninth, Tenth, Eleventh, and Twelfth Chakras

There are the external chakras. When I write "external chakras," I mean that these chakras are found to constantly exist outside of the physical body. They are not external to the energy body. Since most of the time, most people think only of their physical body as being what they are / the location that they exist in. It is a comparative description of location to call them external chakras. In fact, they are well within the body if the energy body is recognized as being part of who/what we are. Anyway, I will call them the external chakras, or the eighth to twelfth chakras.

In different trainings that I have taken, they were placed slightly differently. Some trainings put the eighth chakra between the seventh and ninth. In some trainings, there are many various chakras that they talk about. In quantum healing, the five external chakras are taught the way they are because they have shown to be consistently functional in all the people who have learned them this way. Some systems teach elaborate systems of alignments between the chakras. If you have had various trainings that place or use them differently, try this system as it is taught and then see how it intermingles with, or gives you more perspective on, the other teachings or not.

Some teachings call the eighth, ninth, tenth, eleventh, and twelfth chakras the soul chakras. So I may refer to them by number or as the soul chakras or the external chakras. They don't have colors attached to them in most teachings that I have encountered. Maybe because most people who work with the external chakras can see in energy and maybe because they are not so associated with the way that we see in the physical. If you do place or project colors into these chakras, it will affect the vibration of the chakras, but we won't get into that now. For now, we will merely work to build a relationship with these five chakras and bring them into our conscious control.

To develop a relationship with the chakras is the key. To do so requires a raised vibration or the ability to have a highly developed sensitivity to subtle energy. So we will work to develop and foster the ability to do both at the same time with the quantum healing techniques. Before we do the exercise to build awareness of these five chakras and bring them under the control of our conscious minds, we will get a little more info about them and the other chakras that we will be working with.

**12th chakra**

 **11th chakra**

 **10th chakra**

 **9th chakra**

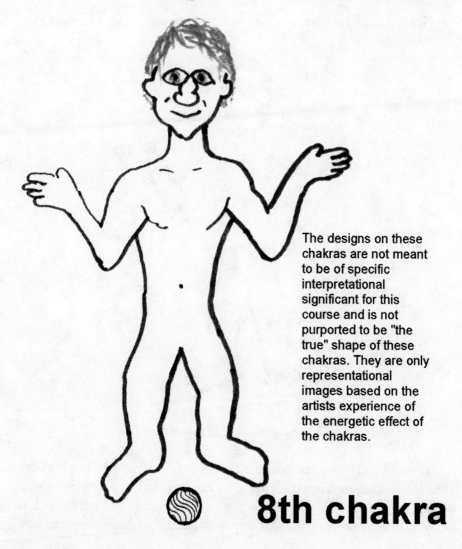

The designs on these chakras are not meant to be of specific interpretational significant for this course and is not purported to be "the true" shape of these chakras. They are only representational images based on the artists experience of the energetic effect of the chakras.

**8th chakra**

Whatever you want to call them is OK. When you get to know them, you will like them.

The last set of chakras that we will work with is the minor chakras. They are talked about and used in some Taoist teachings. They are in the limbs, at the feet/ankles, knees, hips, hands/wrists, elbows, and shoulders. There are a lot of them—twelve. The arm's chakras are in the arms, and the leg's chakras are in the legs. The energetics of these chakras are not as strong/intense/noticeable as the other chakras, so we do them last when our awareness and sensitivity is greatest.

## Minor Chakra Chart ~ Arms Chakras and Legs Chakras

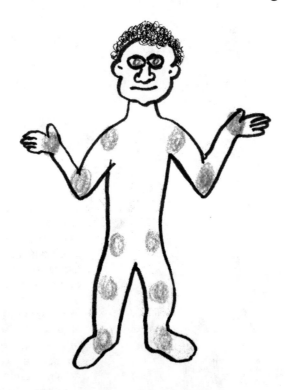

*relativity of chakras at appendix #4*

To build a relationship with your chakras is easy. First, we will work with your internal seven chakras. Starting at the first chakra at the perineum, bring your awareness to that area and sense what energy you feel there. It is a subtle energy that may not have any distinguishable shape or describable feeling. In order to make it easier to find and work with the chakras, you can first clear and increase your energy with the white, red, and pink aura cleaning method described earlier and do the six six quantum healing breath while spiraling your waves of awareness and spinning the energy balls in your hands. By combining these two methods, your awareness/sensitivity to energy is increased enough to make finding/sensing your chakras easy.

Once you have found the energy of your first chakra, have it accumulate into a sphere about the size of an orange or cantaloupe. Once you have accumulated the chakra into that shape, have it spin. The direction that you choose for it to spin is not important; any direction is good. It is not spiraling; it is spinning. If at first it hesitates to do as you direct it, try communicating other ways. Some people tell their chakras, others ask, some intend, some visualize, and some imagine the changes in shape and direction of spinning. At first I told/intended; then later I found it was easier to get them to follow if I "asked them to" be a shape and spin one way or another. Now that I have a good relationship with them, any manner of directing them works well.

People find their chakras in all variations of sizes and shapes. Other modalities teach people to put their chakras into many various shapes and do various activities with them. None of them are wrong, just different. There are many teachings about the use and utility of your chakras that are practically useful, and they do what they are said to if practiced correctly. *Many of them have some precautions and have direct recommendations of correct use.* My experience has shown me that it is safe to follow teachings, and once you come to understand them, use the practices correctly, but that the precautions are there for good reason. But like I did, many years ago, you may have to learn the hard way. Yes, I have thrown caution to the wind and paid the price a few times. It was many years ago, and each time, it took a long time to fully recover my energy and understand what had happened. Believe me, the progress is much faster by following the teachings and precautions and staying in integrity.

Your chakras are energy events that are not governed by the same laws of physics that we believe govern matter as we understand it. You are the true and only master of your chakras, so they will move to any shape or size and spin or spiral and suck or spew any way that you direct them to. Whatever they do is going to have an effect on your perceptions and your ability to maintain the correct functioning of your body's tissue. That is why I like to be conscious of mine and have a good working relationship with them so that I can keep them functioning to my benefit. To have them functioning in correct alignment so that they raise your vibration to the highest level is the goal of the methods taught in quantum healing.

After you have accumulated/shaped the first chakra into a sphere and gotten it spinning, intend that it continues to do so in that position and move to the next. Find the second chakra, have it form a sphere the same size, and then get it to spin in any direction that you choose. They can spin in the same or different directions. Sometimes, having your chakras spinning in different directions is better than having them all spin the same way. Once the second chakra is spinning, and you have intended it to continue to do so, then do the same thing with the third. Continue to do the same for the fourth, fifth, sixth, and seventh. When you have gone through all seven internal chakras and all seven internal chakras are spinning, bring your attention to how the energy balls around your hands feel. See if you can sense a difference in how it feels with the seven chakras spinning to how it feels without the seven chakras spinning. The first time you do this exercise, you may be too busy with the chakras to notice the shift in the subtle feeling that you perceive from the energy balls around your hands as they spin on the exhale of your six six breaths while you work within the pink energy field that you have filled your aura with. So do it three times to get familiar with the technique and the various sensations.

It is important to do this exercise fully now so that you will be comfortable to combine the next steps with it soon. So take your time and work this practice spinning one chakra at a time and leaving it spinning as you go to the next and get it spinning, and then when they are all spinning, go back through them all one at a time and get them to spin faster. Next, go through them and have them change the direction of the spinning in each chakra, either one at a time or all at once.

Now that you have a bit of a relationship with the seven chakras, it is time to work with the colors in them. First, we will put the color from one chart into the chakras and see how that feels. Then we will go back to clear and put the other set of colors in our chakras and see if we can describe the difference. Then we will do some exercises to build our relationship deeper and refine our sensitivity to the subtle variations in the sensations of the energetics that we create.

One color set                          the other color set

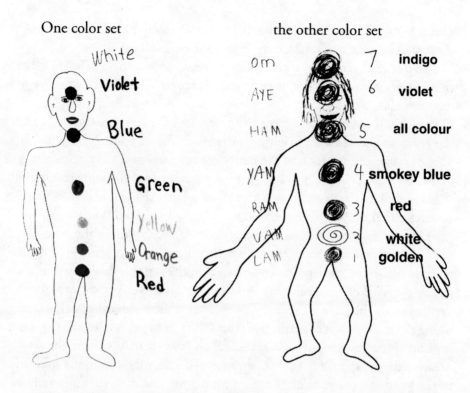

Ya, some folks say I got the colors off shade a little from how I describe the colors to be, but I say, "That's OK 'cuz you can color your chakras any color you want anyway."

The best explanation that I can give for everyone to do this exercise is the answer I got from a student in one of my seminars. In that seminar, one woman who was well versed in energy work seemed perplexed about why there was the other color chart and why we would want to put other colors in our chakras. I explained as I have earlier that the chakra colors change with our moods, thoughts, and actions as well as other possible influences and then asked Rick (another student that was taking the class) what he sees when he looks at people's chakra colors. Rick is very clairvoyant and has been all of his life. He supported what I had said and went on to say that sometimes people's chakra colors change as they go about their business. He gave an example of watching people's chakras at a mall and seeing them with distinct colors in their chakras before walking up and talking to each other and noticing the colors, and sometimes the positions too, change during the conversation that they share; and then when they walk away from each other, their chakra colors were quite different from when he first observed them. He went on to add a confirmation that many people have colors in their chakras that don't match the either of the charts at all.

To put a color into your chakra is simple. Once you have it into a sphere shape and it is spinning, just intend that color to be in your chakra or imagine that the chakra is that color or visualize that color as brightly filling the chakra or ask the chakra to glow the color. Use the same method to adjust the color to the hue and brightness that you like. If you have any doubts about your ability to achieve the perfect shade in your chakra according to the shade as you choose it to be, then just imagine that you can achieve that shade and then imagine that you are achieving that shade and then continue to intend that your chakra be filled with that shade until it is.

Once you have all seven chakras colored according to the first chart you choose, continue with the six six breath for several breaths to notice anything that you can about any variance in the sensations that you notice in the energy balls around your hands and then in your body and overall. Next, put all the chakras back to clear. Then follow the other color chart, filling the chakras one at a time with the colors from that chart. Do the same sensing of the energy balls around your hands while maintaining the six six breath with the spiraling waves of awareness on the inhales and the spinning in the hands on the exhale. After you have done this long enough to notice if you are sensing a variation in the feeling of the energetics, you can stop. I suggest that you introduce and feel the effects of each color system three times, one and then the other, before you make a final determination of what the differences are. As at first, many people don't notice any difference; but after they perform the exercise a few times, many of them seem to develop a keen sensitivity of the various sensations that are presented from the variance in the energetics on all levels.

In the class, there is an advanced exercise that we perform next. It is necessary to be comfortable with the changing of chakra colors while maintaining the six six breath to perform this one, but so far everyone has succeeded, so I know that you can too. It is a little more in-depth than the other ones. Basically, you will fill the chakras with the colors that you choose from one chart or the other. Next, you will allow one chakra at a time to glow, or radiate, out the color that you have placed in it. When it is radiating out the color or glowing, it will not be leaking or sending out any of its chakra energy, only the light vibration of the color will be projected in all directions from the chakra. Just the color shines brightly around the chakra. And as your spiraling waves of awareness strobe past the chakras, the waves of awareness will be tinted by the glowing color of the chakra, or you could say that the waves of awareness pick up on and mimic the hue of the glowing color of the chakra as it passes. The hue or tint is carried to the energy balls with each wave as you inhale and is spun in the energy balls as you exhale. As the tinted energy balls spin during your exhale, notice if you can sense a subtle, or not subtle, variation in the sensation of the energy balls. After several breaths, the color in the chakra is stopped from radiating out, and one breath with its six waves of awareness is taken without any color radiating out from any chakra so that the waves and the tint of the energy ball go back to untinted/clear. Then you follow the same routine with the next chakra.

After doing this running of the *mimic of the chakra colors* to the hands one at a time, you do them all at once. Have all the chakras glow or radiate out their perspective colors all at the same time and allow the waves of awareness to be tinted by all the colors so that all the colors are spinning in the hands all at the same time. Notice how this affects the sensation of energy in those balls. Then go back to clear in the chakras before doing the same thing with the other color chart. After going through both charts two or three times in this manner, take a little time to reflect on the experience. What did it feel like in each stage with each color?

Next, you can start to get familiar with the five external chakras. To do that, let the seven internal chakras go back to normal or dormant. I don't like the term "dormant," but it seems to get the idea of no conscious activity across to almost everyone, so I use it. I don't believe that chakras are ever truly dormant, so this word is not the best description of what is meant here. What is meant is stop them from spinning and allow them to relax or transform into other shapes, remove conscious control from them. Then stand up and reinitiate the white, red, and pink to clear your energy and aura and start the six six spiraling breaths with the spinning on the exhales. Bring your attention to the eighth chakra, in the area about eight to ten inches below your feet. The eighth chakra is usually in the ground, but because it is an energy event rather than a physical aspect of our body, being in the ground is not a problem for it. Feel for the energetic that is there and accumulate it into a sphere; have it spin and intend that it continues to spin there. The ninth chakra is next about eight to ten inches above your head. Feel for the energetic that is there and accumulate it into a sphere, have it spin and intend that it continues to spin there. And so on to the twelfth chakra.

After or during doing this, you may notice that this was/is easier than when you started with the internal seven chakras. This is both because you have gained sensitivity, skill, confidence, and familiarity with subtle energetics and because you have risen in vibration so that you are more in tune with energy, more energized, and thus more able to work with energy. Once you get chakras eight to twelve spinning, continue with the six six breath with the spiraling waves of awareness on the inhales and the spinning in the hands on the exhale for several breaths, focusing on how the energetics around your hands feel and see if you can discern a variance in them. Next, while you continue with the soul chakras spinning and the six six breath, bring your attention to how you feel overall: how you feel in relationship to the room, how your physical body feels, how the things/objects/people in the room feel in relation to you, how you feel in relation to the things around the room. Then bring the soul chakras back to their previous (not under conscious control / dormant) condition.

Activate only chakras one to seven and do the six six breath with the spiraling waves of awareness on the inhales and the spinning in the hands on the exhale for several breaths, focusing on how the energetics around your hands feel and see what you can discern in their energetic. Then breathe, bring your attention to how you feel overall: how you feel in relationship to the room, how your physical body feels, how the things/objects/people in the room feel in relation to you, how you feel in relation to the things around the room.

Do this comparison two or three times for your personal benefit and practice. Then get all twelve chakras spinning at the same time and do it again like that. See what the difference is. Try it again and see if you notice anything more. I always like the feedback from the group after these exercises. The words are sometimes different, but the description of the effects are always the same. I won't share it here so that you can have the experience. I will talk about it later.

The next step is to align the chakras into their internal positions. This takes place in two stages in the class. First, we bring in the external chakras; then, we build a relationship with the minor chakras and incorporate them into the alignment. The vibrational shift that takes place with the internal positions makes it easier to bring the minor chakras into our awareness and to realign them. Various trainings that I have taken have slight variations on how the external chakras align within the body. I have worked with them in a trial and error manner to discern what the differences are and what the variation in effect is. I have done this experimenting alone and with colleagues to determine what works best, and I believe I have found something special. What I found is that the system of alignment that is taught here is naturally found by everyone who takes the class and that they all become comfortable with it after a very few alignments. Most people have felt great with it the first time, but a few folks found the unfamiliarity more noticeable than anything else, at least the first time they did it. A couple of people said that they preferred their old alignment at first but didn't mention it again as we continued with the other work that followed. One person stated that she had two eleventh chakras in the internal position and was uncomfortable with congealing them into one, but she was comfortable with all the internal positions. I may not be the best one to state the result as I keep this alignment most of the time, and I am used to it, so I don't truly notice the benefits as being anything more than normal now. The reason that I started to maintain the fourteen internal positions of my chakras spinning was an elevated sense of clarity and awareness that was accompanied by a calm, stable feeling in my core.

To achieve the internal alignment, you stand up and bring in the white and the red to fill yourself and your aura with the effervescent pink, perform the six six breath with the spiraling waves of awareness on the inhale and the spinning in the hands on the exhale, activate all twelve chakras by getting them to form spheres and spin, and then invite the soul chakras into their internal positions. The eighth chakra fits about halfway between the second and third. This is slightly beneath the navel. The ninth chakra has a natural seat about halfway between the third and fourth chakras at about the level of the solar plexus. The tenth chakra fits at the bottom of the throat below and partly shares space with the fifth chakra. The eleventh chakra sits between the sixth and seventh, about in the middle of the brain. The twelfth sits halfway out of the top of your head, partly superimposed over the seventh. As you bring them into their internal alignment places, you allow/get them to move up and down and side to side and back and forth to find their most comfortable correct position. When all twelve of them are in their most comfortable correct internal positions, you intend that they continue to spin there and continue with the six six breath with spiraling waves of awareness on the inhale and the spinning in the hands on the exhale while you build relationships with the minor chakras.

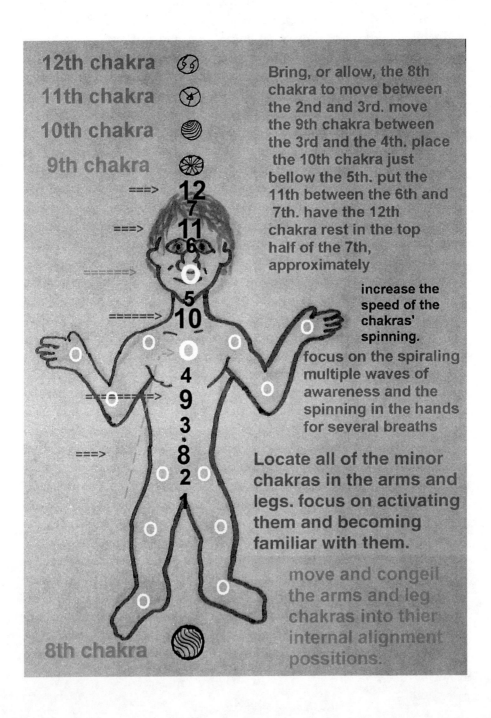

12th chakra

11th chakra

10th chakra

9th chakra

===> 12
7
===> 11
6
=======> O
5
=======> 10
O O O
4
==O==> 9
3
·8
===> 2 O
1

8th chakra

Bring, or allow, the 8th chakra to move between the 2nd and 3rd. move the 9th chakra between the 3rd and the 4th. place the 10th chakra just bellow the 5th. put the 11th between the 6th and 7th. have the 12th chakra rest in the top half of the 7th, approximately

increase the speed of the chakras' spinning.

focus on the spiraling multiple waves of awareness and the spinning in the hands for several breaths

Locate all of the minor chakras in the arms and legs. focus on activating them and becoming familiar with them.

move and congeil the arms and leg chakras into thier internal alignment possitions.

To build a conscious relationship with the minor chakras while having the twelve chakras in the internal position is easy. While maintaining the red, white, and pink and six six breath, you turn your attention to the minor chakras. First, you bring your attention to your feet and notice the energetic there. It will feel similar to that of the other chakras but not precisely the same and not as intense, or should I say less noticeable. Then you accumulate them into spheres and have them spin. You could do them one at a time or both at once. Next, you do the same thing for the knee's chakras, then the hip's chakras; and then the hand's, elbow's, and shoulder's chakras. Once you have them all spinning, ask the legs chakra to come up to the space between the heart and tenth chakras and have them converge to occupy the same space and all spin in that one space. They can merge and spin as one or spin in various directions all within the same space to make one sphere with its center about halfway between the heart and tenth chakras. Have the congealed legs chakra move up and down and side to side and back and forth to find its most comfortable correct position and then do the same for the arms chakra. The position for the arms chakra is between the fifth and sixth chakras, approximately at the back of the mouth. Like with the leg's, the arm's chakras are located in the hand/wrists, elbows and shoulders. They are similar in sensation to the leg's chakras. Locate them, have them spin in their locations where you found them, and then have them all converge on a space between the fifth and sixth chakras, approximately at the back of the mouth. Allow the arms chakra to spin as one or all converged exactly in the same position to form one sphere. Have the arms chakra then move up and down, back and forth, and side to side to find its most comfortable correct position between the fifth and sixth chakras. Then have the twelfth chakra adjust to superimpose itself completely in the same place as the seventh chakra if it is not already there and notice if you feel a shift take place in your energy.

With all thirteen chakra positions spinning in the internal alignment, continue doing the six six breath and spinning the energy balls in your hands. Notice how the energy balls feel as they spin in/around your hands. Notice how you feel in relation to the energy balls. Notice how you feel in relation to your physical body. Notice how you feel in relation to your energy body/aura and how you feel in relation to the room around you and to the area around the room. Spend a few moments working the six six breath and feeling the various aspects of this exercise. In the classes, it often takes students several times of doing this before they notice all the subtle differences. The feedback that I have gotten back from them has always been similar in the descriptions of the energetics that they have experienced.

To try to explain what happens with this fourteen chakra positions to anyone who has not explored this alignment is like trying to describe a scent to someone with no sense of smell. To explain the result of what happens, it is fair to say that it consolidates the relationships that you have built with your chakras. This consolidation allows you to experience all the benefits of your activated chakras without being distracted by the benefit of any individual chakra or group of chakras. By bringing all of your chakras into your conscious awareness, you are more easily able to sustain their activeness, or activated state. The alignment itself does ignite a very subtle shift in your overall energetic, but many people don't notice this change in their energetic until they explore it more deeply.

I have had several people tell me many months after my classes that they have noticed real changes in the awareness of my students. They have told me about changes in attitudes, conscious behavior, health, demeanor, vitality, as well as the changes in the energetics of my students. I have seen some of these changes too. Personalities of the students are all individual, so results do vary, but the changes do occur and can be seen in their energetics. It is hardest to notice changes in ourselves because as we look out at the world we see it from our own perspective, and as our perspective changes, it looks to us like the world has changed—not us. As we rise in vibration and increase our abilities in awareness, we are able to see, feel, understand, and hear things that were hidden from our view before. As our actions are chosen and done in the present moment, we most closely identify with how we are rather than how we were, and others hold the memory of how we were (from their perspective as observers). So without much understanding of how we are, others compare our new behaviors with our older ones and often judge us as having changed some. If the changes that they notice are in alignment with their values and interests, many say it is a good change; and if they notice changes that diverge from their interests and values, it is likely to be described as a bad change, or a change for the worst. We are who we are, and we are all different; our true value and identity is not determined by other's opinions, but we can take a reading on our progress and direction from the feedback of those who choose to judge us.

For several years, I have been exploring my relationships with my chakras in several various modalities of energy training. What I have realized is that once you have developed a relationship with your chakras you can move them anywhere you want to and form them into any shape you like. But just like the color of your internal seven chakras have an effect on your perceptions, the energetic that any of your chakras pick up as they interact with other energies have an effect on how they affect your energy body and physical body. You can move your chakras out of your body to any distant location, but what happens to it, there will/may have permanent effects on you energetically.

To explain the seriousness of maintaining correct energetic balance and "health" of your chakra system, let me use examples from other energy systems. If you have a single block in a single meridian, you may notice sensitivity at the location of that energy blockage on that meridian, and you will experience the dysfunction of the tissue that is supplied with chi by that meridian. The tender point on the meridian may go unnoticed for some time before the malfunctioning tissue gets your attention. If your aura has some stuff (anything that is not your own energy) in it, it will slowly work through the layers of the aura and affect your physical health, thoughts, and attitudes. For instance, you can always see tiny spots in an aura before and during a cold or flu. If you clean the aura of the spots before the cold or flu starts to have a physical effect on the person's body, they don't get the cold or flu; if you wait until after the cold or flu symptoms have affected the person, the clearing of the spots from the aura will diminish the symptoms but not always completely relieve the cold or flu. This is because after the energy of the cold or flu has entered the physical body it starts to disrupt the balance and flow of chi in your meridian and balance of chi in your organs. Any incorrect energetic in one or more of your chakras will diminish your ability to become who you truly are or should I say prevent you from experiencing your life as fully as you deserve to.

The seven internal chakras have a direct relationship with the functioning of your endocrine system and an energetic relationship with your personality development. The outer five chakras have a direct relationship with your abilities to relate to everything other than your own physical body, and your minor chakras of the arms and legs have a direct relationship with your abilities to interact with your physical as well as energetic surroundings. They all have important parts to play in the maintaining of your ability to experience life in the physical and energetic world that we live in. If you choose to do various things with your chakras after this course, you will have the training to understand a little about how you are affecting yourself.

I suggest that you take the time to asses your relationship with your chakras before and after doing this and other energy work training or experimenting. I also suggest that you be cautious if you do choose to do any experimenting with your chakras. If you are the curious type like me, it may be in your best interest to learn from those who have gone before you before risking peril needlessly. I have studied many paths before putting together this shortcut to elevated awareness, and it has been an interesting and exciting learning journey. I still take courses on modalities that I find interesting whenever I can. After decades of learning, I have come to understand the deepest meaning of the proverb "You don't know what you don't know," and it has become my guide to wisdom.

With the shift in your vibration that takes place utilizing the training in this book, you can gain tremendous insight to how life force energy works. There are many other trainings that teach about energy in different ways and various aspects of energy and how to move it and use it. Some are healthful, and some can be harmful. Never be scared to learn a modality but always be cautious and mindful of what is happening to your own energy and your energetics when you participate in practices that are new to you. Once you become familiar with a new way of being with your energy and energetic, that familiarity usually gives a sense of comfort. Before accepting a sense of comfort as an improvement check to see if you have gained any abilities or skills of sensitivities or if you feel the bonds of attachments or the restrictions of barriers and beliefs are not supported by experience. Be true to who you are. Knowledge is good, and truth brings enlightenment.

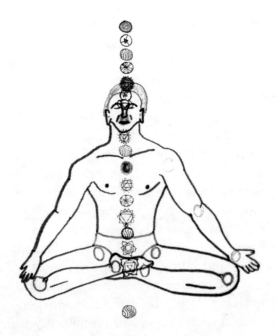

## Chapter Five

# *Healing Methods and Practice*

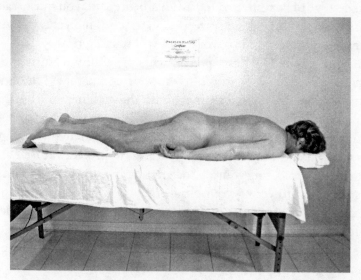

**Note:** It is not necessary to have your clients naked, but don't be shocked if you encounter a client or two who choose to get naked before climbing on the table. Remember that it is OK to cover them up with a sheet or blanket, and thus, it is good to have one handy.

In this chapter, the practical and theoretical as well as the intellectual, spiritual, social, benevolent, and business aspects of healing will be covered in a holistic context. The reason for this is that they are all part of the one issue of providing a quality healing experience for your clients. Ya see, if your client thinks of you as anything less than a competent professional practitioner of what you have trained in, they will disrespect you in some little way that will/may undermine your ability to help them and others. In our society, people are trained to think that they must pay for value and that they will get what they pay for, if they are lucky. Many people are also taught double standards like nothing of value is available for free—and they should not have to pay full price for anything that they can get cheep. This particular double standard leads to them asking for a reduced rate or free introduction to your services, which, if granted, in turn causes them to disrespect you and your services because they see you as needy for clients to practice on and not recognizing your own offered rate as being the fair rate for your work/services. Well, not everyone is like this, but those who are seldom become return clients who are willing to pay and refer their friends. In a nutshell, the service you provide when you do this work is of great value, and you deserve to be respected for it. That being said, you must realize that this work deserves to be done correctly. "Correctly" indicates that there are ethics involved in this field of work, so I will start there.

Ethically, it is prudent as a person with the ability to sustain a higher than normal vibration to do so as often as possible and for as long as you can each time you do. This is in alignment with the oath near the beginning of the book. It is also ethical to respect yourself as a person who has expended effort to improve yourself with the end result being that you are capable of helping yourself and others and that you need to protect yourself and your ability to do so. Protecting yourself socially and intellectually is as important in our society as protecting yourself energetically. To do this, simply treat your training as professional and act accordingly. When someone asks a doctor for medical advice on the bus or at a party, the doctor almost always suggests that they call the office and book an appointment. Same with a lawyer, an engineer, or any other professional.

Once when I was teaching a seminar at my old Qigong master's studio, his neighbor confronted my students and me as we were going out for lunch. He was mocking my old master and me for doing energy work and at the same time suggesting that I should be able to heal him of his health issues. I told him that he could call me to book a session if he was serious and gave him a card. He looked a little shocked and asked me if I did it for a living and asked how much I charged. When I told him my rate, he looked at me with a considerable increased amount of respect and failed to say another word; he went back into his house. I didn't ever hear from him to book a session, but he didn't bother me or my students anymore. Remember that you have got nothing to prove to anyone and that you are doing what you have chosen to do. Therefore, it is intrinsically the correct thing for you to be doing, and act accordingly. This will gain you the respect that you deserve.

During that episode with my old Qigong master's neighbor, I continued to hold my energy at a high vibrational state and noticed how he was energetically trying to disrupt my emotional balance with his mocking and body gestures. I simply witnessed his antics but noticed how my students felt uncomfortable with his words and gestures. Basically, he was attempting to bully us into conforming to his nonbelief in energy work. His attempt to put himself as an authority (in our minds) of what is "real" failed. By simply acting as a professional energy worker and offering him a professional service, I prevented him from perpetrating the harm of humiliation upon my students for following their personal interest in the training that I offer. This example of how easy it is to gain acceptance for what many are coming to respect as important from those who have no understanding or interest in it can be followed by anyone safely and comfortably in any social situation. In our society, if you act professional about anything, you will be accepted as an authority on that topic by most people. The rednecks may not accept the topic of your authority as being relevant, but they will accept that you are the/an authority in that topic.

To start doing a session first you need a client. It can be anyone: yourself, a friend, family member, pet, plant, volunteer, or a paying client. I prefer paying clients. Mostly because I don't like to work for free, but also because they are usually the best clients. People who are willing to pay for your time and effort are usually glad to receive the help that you give them. It is OK to work on people for free if you feel they would benefit from your efforts, but if they refuse your help or say "You can try," you may want to ask yourself why you would bother working on them. If they are not going to welcome and respect the effort of the work that you are going to perform, why would you work to put out that effort? If they are going to be paying you for the work and you are OK working for an ungrateful, overbearing, obnoxious employer or client, then of course, working for pay makes sense. However, if you are not getting paid and your work is not going to be welcomed and respected, you should respect yourself and your capacity to provide a valuable service and refrain from degrading yourself. After all, we all have free will; if someone is choosing to suffer needlessly, who are you to prevent them from following their choice? So a willing client is best.

This leads to the issue of permission. Under spiritual law, we all have the right to accept and/or refuse any energy that is sent from another being. So if you have an unwilling client, they may refuse the energy, and it may bounce back to you. Ya see, there are only two possible destinations for energy to arrive at. It is like the postal service; if the energy that is intended to be delivered to a client is refused, it is returned to the sender. However, unlike the mail, it is returned with an amplified delivery. This is true with hands-on and distance healing. With hands-on healing, you usually are aware if the client is refusing the energy as they are there to talk with you about it. With distance, it is good to ask for permission first. There are times when permission is not necessary. If you have a custodial relationship with any being—meaning that you are the primary caretaker of any life-form that is not mature enough to understand and make decisions concerning their own well-being or is somehow confined or controlled by you so that their survival and well-being is determined by you without their input—then you have a spiritual responsibility to do all that you can to help them, and that includes doing energy work.

Specifically with the quantum healing energy work techniques, if performed as taught, there is virtually no risk to the practitioner if the energy is refused. In fact, for the most part the energy is not being sent to or placed into or upon the client/receiver in a quantum healing session but only put adjacent to them or amid their energetics. The way that quantum healing works is via the simple laws of physics governing resonance and entrainment. As one item resonates at any vibration, it will have an effect of influencing the things near to it toward resonating at the same vibration. The rate of vibration is called relative resonance, and the effect of bringing other forms to resonate at the same frequency is called entrainment. The pluck of a string resonates and brings your eardrum to vibrate at the same rate thus entraining to sense the sound correctly.

Resonance and entrainment—that is what you are doing when you use the quantum healing technique. You raise and sustain your vibration very high and hold that high vibration adjacent to another being until they entrain to the higher vibration. When they do, their physical form recognizes flaws or discrepancies between its design and its actual state and shifts to the correct form. This happens on all physical, emotional, physiological, mental, and energetic levels to varying degrees depending on the individuals involved and the vibrational state reached and entrained to. As you rise in vibration to perform the work, you are already exposing your entire being to the higher vibration, so if the energy is refused, it will not have a significantly different effect than it would have had by simply doing the treatment/session had it been fully received. Technically speaking, you are never intending the QH healing to have an effect directly/specifically, but only to be present for the receiver/client to entrain to and thus respond to according to the design of their own body's/being's design and abilities.

Most clients that come to have a session will expect that you work on them with your hands on their body. This is OK because you have learned to put the energy balls that you can use for the healing effect around your hands. So to get the best and fastest hands on results, simply place one hand on either side of the problem area of the client's body and continue until you feel, or sense, that the two balls of energy have merged through the client to become one connected energetic reaching from one of your hands to the other. Sometimes, clients don't want to be touched. For them, you can hold your hands a short distance off their body and do the same thing and get the same result. There is also a hands-free technique that will be covered on the next pages that is very versatile and easy to perform.

It is always crucial that you specifically ask the client permission to touch them. Even though they may indicate that they will be comfortable with it, it is important to get verbal permission. If you want, you can require written permission; and in some jurisdictions, this may be legally important. It is best to let the client know where you will be touching them because some people have issues with being touched in various places. For instance, I have had people sternly insist that I not touch their ears and another say that they don't like their hands touched and one say to not touch her neck. I have been asked to specifically work on breasts and butts, but I always specifically get permission before touching these areas or any area of a client's body before doing so no matter what they said before they got on the table or on the chair. Most often, if a woman comes for a session for you to work on her breast cancer, she will want you to work on her breast directly. It is not always the case, and it is also not necessary that you put your hand on her breast to do the session.

There is an aspect of being a good practitioner that requires you to do what the client expects from you within the context of the work to a certain extent. For instance, if the client wants you to work hands-on, it is most likely that they will recognize you as a good practitioner if you do work hands-on. Often the client will have some concept of what you as a practitioner will want to or are going to do that is based on another therapy that they have heard about or experienced. That is OK. It may not be accurate, and you must do what you must do to provide the service that you are willing to provide. So be willing to tell the client what your session will consist of. Be willing to be clear with them about what you do and what you won't do. Be professional in your communication with them, but don't necessarily tell them more than they want to hear. For instance, there are some people who may believe that your therapy can help them who would not believe anything that you could tell them about how it works or what you are actually doing. They may be able to believe some of it after having several or many sessions, but if they hear too much too soon, they will never have a second session.

It is never necessary to touch any areas of a client's body that you are not comfortable touching. If your client has prostate cancer or cervical cancer, it is not necessary to get a hand or hands on to, or in to, their genitals or even near them. If you put one hand on the side of each hip, the prostate or cervix will be between your hands, and you will be able to give a direct session to the area that the client is concerned about. This is effective and comfortable for both most clients and most practitioners.

It is important to have your massage table or chair or other work situation arranged so that you can be comfortable while doing the sessions. It is good to consider how you will sit or stand before you situate the client for the session and how you will deal with disruptions like the phone or the door, etc., before you start a session. It is best if you are ready to do whatever you need to do to proceed with a session showing confidence and professionalism from the start to the finish. Also, if they are paying, it is good to be ready to give them a receipt.

Part of being a good practitioner is keeping a record of the session. In the classes, I always have the participants record each session. They take the name of the client, the date, and time of the session, the main issue worked on, and the results as they noticed and as they asked the clients for feedback and record the results of the client according to what the client said they noticed during and after the session. This is often helpful in future session for many reasons. (*a*) If you don't see a client for a few years, you have a record of what the session was and who they are—you know they will remember the details of the session if they are calling for another one, so it is good to read the file before you see them again. (*b*) Sometimes a client will report good results after a session and forget about it before the next session, so if they call to cancel and say that "it did nothing for me," you can remind them of what they reported as a result and often save the session and build a good relationship with a client that turns into future referrals. (*c*) When the client sees you taking notes in the session, they feel like you take their concerns seriously and notice your professionalism. (*d*) If they mention you or your therapy to another practitioner who calls you to confer about the client, you have something to refer to when you talk to them. (*e*) In the rare event that a claim is made against you, you have a record of what was done in the session, which makes whatever you say about it more credible. Truly though, to get a good result, you need only do the energy work; but in our postmodern society, these other considerations are real and important.

The actual technique to perform quantum healing is quite easy and straightforward. After you ask the client what they want you to work on and get them situated so that you can be comfortable while you are doing the work, you can start. The first thing that needs to be done, of course, is the white, red, and pink practice of filling and cleaning your natural human life force energy in your body and aura. Next, you forget any bad stuff that you may have heard about the client and create an image of their perfection to hold in your mind until after the session is over. Then you activate your chakras and guide them into the thirteen chakra positions. Then you get specific permission to put your hands wherever you will want to put them while you are treating the client (performing the quantum healing session). Then you do the multiple spiraling waves of awareness on each inhale and spin the energy balls around your hands as you exhale while you have your hands on the client. Ya, that's it. It is a big chapter to say that, ah?

As you are doing the session, you may get an intuition to move your hands to another or several other positions on the client. If you are not sure if the client will be OK with you moving your hands, ask them about the new locations before or as you are moving your hands to them. While doing quantum healing, your intuition is usually the best way to determine what to do next. If your client is accustomed to you following a specific pattern of hand placements or you have told them that you will be following a certain procedure, then it is best/good to follow the expected format.

It is good to keep the client involved in the decisions during a session as it gives them the feeling of control in their process of healing. It helps put the concept into their unconscious mind that they are responsible for their well-being. That is why in quantum healing, the terminology is that the client is the healer, and the practitioner is the facilitator of the healing. If the client is informed that it is their body responding to the energy presented in the session, and thus that it is their body that actually does the healing, then their unconscious mind gets the message that *it* is responsible for the results of the session. This message also allows the unconscious mind to bring forth the truth that the individual is responsible for their health.

Accurately, the client is doing the healing within this modality as the intense high vibrational energy balls created adjacent to the client's body do not do the healing themselves directly. In fact, the healing takes place as the client's body entrains to that higher vibration and thereafter. Sometimes the client's body continues to correct itself for days and weeks after a single session. I have had some clients claim no result after a session and phone me up days later to tell me all their improvements and how they incrementally showed up in stages as time passed.

If you have more than one practitioner doing quantum healing on a client, the results are sometimes more noticeable. If both, or all, practitioners are doing the same breath, chakra, spiral patterns, then the energetic that they each are creating is similar enough so that it entrains the client as one, and usually the client only will notice the energy affecting them in one way at a time. If the practitioners are doing various breath and chakra and spiral patterns, then the client may notice several different shifts taking place at the same time at varied rates in different parts of their body.

The length of a session can be as short as eight minutes to get a noticeable results most of the time. I like to give a twenty or thirty minute sessions. As that gives ample time for the client to say what ever they want to say, to do the quantum healing, record the session and book a time for the next session if appropriate. Some clients think that a longer session is better. I do allow them to book them, but longer sessions are not always better. I have found that with two-hour sessions, often clients forget how they felt before they came to the session and claim that they got no result. The first few times this happened, I was shocked and confused. I watched the pattern and analyzed what was occurring and realized that with a very long successful session the client would shift so far, so many times they find a new level of awareness about themselves, which is separate from the awareness that they had at the start of the session. The result is a comfort with the results of the sessions, which leaves them familiar with the new way of feeling to the extent that their mind simply accepts that they have been feeling that way for a long while.

When a client hobbles in and has a long list of complaints before the session and states that they feel great after the session with a statement like "I feel good, I have no problems, my body is doing great, I don't know why I came here today" and then they walk out with a bounce in their step and cancel their next appointment, I find myself with mixed feelings. After these things have happened to me, I usually feel good about the work that I am doing but worried for the future of my practice. I find that when people get results that are too good to believe, they seldom come back or give referrals. If they do give extreme results referrals, people are not likely to take them seriously anyway. So I like to book shorter sessions and have them come a few times. But it is fun to work very diligently giving long sessions and seeing some great results.

## Distance Healing

Once you have become comfortable with the thirteen chakra positions with the six six breath, it is time to start to utilize the techniques practically in more ways. It is as easy to do quantum healing from a distance as it is with your hands on the client. Sometimes hands-on healing is more appropriate, and sometimes distance healing is more appropriate. If the client is new to the idea that energy work can have a real effect on them, it may be best to start with hands-on healing. Or if the client wants or needs some human contact, it may be best to start with hands-on healing. However, if the client is across the room or across the nation, distance quantum healing is just as fast and effective as hands-on healing.

In many modalities of energy work that include distance healing, there are various methods to achieve distance healing. Basically, they all come down to the same thing. Either you create an image of the client and deliver the healing energy to that image, or you send the energy directly to the actual client. First, we will use the created image style; then later we will do the distance-covering method. Both are as effective, and both are easy to do, only the technique is different.

To create an image, you can make a doll, use a teddy bear, imagine the person full size, hold their picture, have some hair or saliva from them, know their name and location, or any other way of identifying that you intend the energy to be directed to them. For our purposes, because of the method that we use in quantum healing, we will create a small image with our minds of the client to receive the healing energy and hold that small image in our hands. Imagine or visualize a miniature-scale image of the client in each hand. You can do one hand first or both at once. Have the images small enough so that they can comfortably stretch out or sit up in your hand when you close your hands around them. Have one in each hand and each hand gently closed so that the image is capsuled within the space between your fingers and palm. Make sure that the image is small enough that it is not being squashed by your hand. It may sound weird, but the comfort of the client is as important in a distance healing as in a hands-on healing. To do the distance healing, you bring the energetic to your hands just the same as you would to do a hands-on healing. If your client is sensitive and your hands are squeezing the image you have of them, they will feel the pressure. I have had many students say that they feel the energetic of the distance healing more intensely than the hands-on healings.

Before actually doing a distance healing, it is prudent to ask permission to do so. Having permission or not will not change the energetic that you create and provide for the client, but it can allow for a significantly different result from the session. If you do not have permission, you do not know that the client is willing to receive the energy. Under spiritual law, they have the right of refusal. This means that they can choose to not accept the energetic that you are sending them. They do not have to understand what you are doing but simply decide that they do not want that energy that is coming at them, and by stating in thought or words that they refuse it, the energy that you are sending them is returned. The return system is absolute in that the original sender is the only place that it will be sent back to. The amplitude/intensity/strength of the energetic is amplified/increased significantly, and any intention or "wish" attached to the energetic may well be twisted or interpretatively modified according to the various circumstances of the situations involved. In addition to this truth, it is best to have permission because it is rude in the world of psychics to send energy to those who have not given you permission.

I have friends who always feel almost any energy that is sent to them. They immediately can read what the energy is, who sent it, what the feelings and intentions of the sender are, and where the sender is and who is with them. They have the right of refusal or can accept the energy. My friends with this sensitivity are kind people, but I have met others with such sensitivity that are not so kind. Being energetically rude won't make you any friends. Besides, if a potential client or old friend or family member or stranger refuses your offer of help, what gives you the right to impose it upon them? If you can't ask them in person or on the phone, e-mail, etc., you can ask your guides or ask their spirit or higher self. Or at the risk of being rude, you can send it, and it will be refused if they don't want it. There are a few situations where it is not necessary to ask permission. If you are the guardian or custodian of a child or infant or any other being (plant, pet, etc.) and thus you are responsible for the safety and survival of the being at the time, you have a spiritual obligation to do whatever you can to maintain there well-being. In this situation, you are responsible to provide energy assistance to them as best you can. So if it is your own child or a child has been left in your care—for the time that that child is in your care—you have a spiritual responsibility to do the energy work for them and do not have to ask permission. If a child is left in your care, that responsibility ends when its guardian/parent retrieves the child back to their own care, and then it is correct to ask them permission if you want to provide energy work to the child.

For people that are preverbal, the asking for energy assistance or energy healing may be a stare in your eyes with the look of "HELP!" I sometimes see this from infants/ babies and toddlers. When I look at them staring into my eyes, it is deliberate and focused and sometimes from a significant distance. It sometimes seems like they are actually struggling to get my attention by stretching to look past the person who is holding them. When this occurs, I look at the energies around the little beings. Their auras are usually covered with "stuff" that is not of them. Most, if not all, infants are very psychic. They can communicate in thought (telepathy) with those who care to interact with them telepathically. Their intellect is often not well developed, so they are not that interesting to most adults who are telepathic. But they can tell who is able to clean the stuff off them, and they may ask you to do it for them if they see that your aura is clean. That asking with that focused stare into the depths of your mind through your eyes is permission to do so. They almost always seem to stop staring as soon as I get their aura cleaned up. If you want to risk being called a freak, you can talk to their parents about it. I never do.

The next concept of importance here is clarity of energetic. If you think that you know what is best for a client, then you may be correct, but more likely, you are just arrogant. At times, we all believe that we know just what people need. Medically speaking, the Mayo Clinic (one of the most prestigious clinics in North America) has been shown from autopsy results to have been inaccurate in diagnosis a good portion of the time. As a doctor of Chinese medicine, I have learned both Western medical and traditional Chinese medicine diagnosis procedures and techniques. I have become good enough to realize that a diagnosis that is 80 percent accurate is considered very good in the medical industry and often gets good results. This means that 20 percent of the information that was taken from the client is not part of the explanation of what is actually happening with the client according to the practitioner, and that practitioner believes he/she can give a beneficial therapy for sure. I have found both that very often the information collected from the client is inaccurate and that practitioners do make errors in judgment. This often leads to therapy that is marginally useful or misses the mark completely. As a result, hearsay information about a client's condition is worse than a bad guess.

If you add any hope, wish, intention, visualization for specific correction, or change to the energy that you send them, you may not actually be giving them any benefit whatsoever from that effort. And if they happen to refuse the therapy, even for a portion of the session, you may not be pleased with the results/repercussions. The way that quantum healing energy works is that it facilitates a situation where the client's body can utilize the vibrational shift to correct itself where it needs most. Many other healing modalities are concerned with specific manipulations of the client to achieve health for them; but in this modality, you do not have to understand the details of the imbalance, injury, malfunction, deformity, or psychosis. You simply do the technique with an image of them "already being perfect" and allow their body to correct itself.

Once you have the image of the client created twice—*once in each hand*—then imagine that the client (not the image but the client [appendix 1]) is already perfect in every way: perfect physical form, perfect functions of health, perfect emotional health, etc. Fill yourself with the white and red and make the pink fill you and your aura, align the thirteen chakra positions, and start the spiraling waves of awareness running to your hands with the six six breath. Then spin the energy balls around your hands as they host the image/images of the client. While you are doing this the first several times, you may find that it is a lot to do. After you get accustomed to doing it all at once, you will notice that you are able to discern energy shifts taking place in your clients as you are doing the distance healing techniques. They may feel the healing depending on their sensitivity to energy and their ability to recognize those sensations.

The next method of distance healing is what I have come to call the hands-free technique. With this method, you do not run the waves of awareness to the hands. You run the waves of awareness to another location. The chart on the next page is worth a thousand words here.

The spiraling waves of awareness are performed the same way during the six six breath, but when they reach the top of your head, you continue the waves to an external location. While inhaling and feeling the way that your body feels from your feet to your head and then carrying or continuing that momentum to an exterior location several times as you inhale, spin the resulted accumulated energy ball as you exhale. To start with, use your waves of awareness to build a ball about the size of a basketball or volleyball about three feet in front of your face. After you get comfortable with the external ball and spinning it on your exhale, you can start to work with it. Do it with various breath patterns and then incorporate the spiraling waves of awareness.

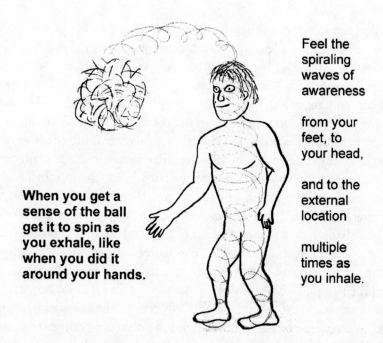

**Feel the spiraling waves of awareness**

**from your feet, to your head,**

**and to the external location**

**multiple times as you inhale.**

**When you get a sense of the ball get it to spin as you exhale, like when you did it around your hands.**

Once you get a sense of the external ball of energy spinning, you can change its size. First, make it smaller in increments until it is the size of a grain of sand. Next, expand the ball every few breaths in increments until it's a size large enough to encompass the whole room. Then bring it back to the basketball size and start to move it around. As you continue to spiral the waves of awareness on the inhale through your mouth of the six six breath, spin the energy ball on the exhale and move it to a new location on every second or third breath. First, move it to your side, then to the other side, then up to the ceiling, then behind you, then behind your feet, then beneath the floor about three feet, then back up in front of you. Next, work with the size again. Make the ball big enough so that you can have it completely around yourself as it spins, then move it to spin around someone else (if you are practicing alone, put it around a large plant or piece of furniture or the fridge).

OK, now we will do two things at once. We will do the waves of awareness to our head and then to our hands and our external location at the same time. You are already capable of both, so instead of splitting the waves into two paths like we have done from the start, we will divide it into three so that the one can go to the external location. Some people have a short challenge with this. Some people started doing several external location balls all at the same time when we first started the hands-free method. It is good to practice this a few times with the spiraling waves and the thirteen chakra positions active. Next, do it with the waves going to the hands and to at least two external-location balls.

When you are working with a client and they are on the table and you are doing a hands-on session, you can use the hands-free balls to increase the intensity in a specific area on the client. For instance, if the client wants you to work on their complexion but you feel that they need some work on their digestion, you can keep your hands on the client's face and put the hands-free balls on or in their stomach and intestines. If the client wants you to do something about their hemorrhoids, you can do hands on their abdomen and hands-free balls in and around their anus, or whatever you and the client are comfortable with. You can also use a hands-free ball around the whole client all through the session to keep clearing the stuff off their aura as you release it from their physical body with balls on/around/in other locations.

You can also use the hands-free ball to change the energy in a room, to charge up your food before you eat it, or for a distance healing. I usually use the hands-free energy balls for distance healing over short distances only, but I believe that the method will work as well over a great distance. It can be combined with distance healing of the other method. If you are giving a distance healing to a client and you believe that there is a part of their body that needs more attention than the rest, you can do a small hands-free energy ball to the tiny images of them that you are holding comfortably in your hands. Make a sand-size hands-free energy ball and place it spinning within the tiny image of your client. Or make several of the tiny balls and sandwich the areas of the images that represent the sections of their body that you feel need the extra attention.

You can also use this or the distance healing method to change the energy in a room or other space or place. By making the hands-free ball big enough to fill a space or room, you can raise the vibration of the entire room all at once. This can also be achieved by holding a tiny image of the room in your hand and doing the energy balls around that hand. You can do this while you are in the space or while you are not in the space. I have used this technique to change the vibe in a nightclub when I wanted to dance. At the time, there was a heavy vibe in the room, and no one was dancing. I did a distance healing on the room for a few moments, and the dance floor started to fill up. The music did not change, but the people in the room showed more smiles, and many of them danced. After about ten to fifteen minutes, the floor started to empty again as the vibe again grew heavy.

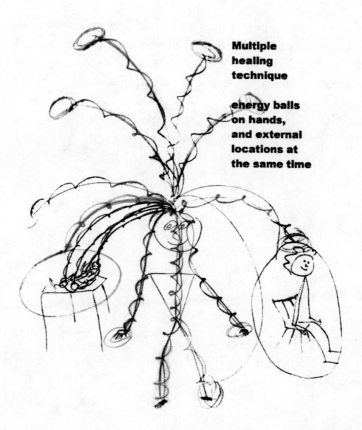

**Multiple
healing
technique**

**energy balls
on hands,
and external
locations at
the same time**

I did the technique several times that evening to get the dance floor filled, and it seemed to work each time. The same technique works at a party where people aren't mingling or any group is acting grumpy. You don't have to be the life of the party, but you can bring life to the party.

This technique can also be used for self-protection. If you are going to be traveling down a path that has a bad vibe, you can give a distance healing on the path and area around it first. If the vibe is still adverse after you give it a distance healing, it may well be time to choose a various path to travel. If you are not sure how to judge the vibe of a path, increase the speed of the spinning of your soul chakras and simply feel/sense/explore with your mind the area of the path.

There are several ways to utilize the hands-free and hands-on. Now that you have the information to achieve these energy-shifting energetics that can have a positive effect on the physical reality, you can start to have fun with them. I hope that you can enjoy this awareness-expanding practice as much as I have. In the level 2 class, we start by working diligently to raise each other's vibration higher than we can achieve on our own with a group activity and work up and sideways from there to achieve a vastly higher and sustainable vibrational state and abilities in awareness. After you become comfortable and familiar with the various applications of the level 1 work, I hope you find a path to level 2 or other similar teachings that will be to your benefit.

# Appendix 1

Here, we are doing two things that may sound like one twice or be confusing. We are doing two different things at the same time or in sequence. One of the things is—either first or second—we create a small image of the client in our hand. Not an image of them being small, but a small image of them. We create that image small enough so that it can comfortably be held in your hand without being pressed into as you close your hand to encapsulate the image. This image is an image of the client as they now exist in the time space reality that we dwell in. The other image that we hold of the client is the image of perfection. This is the second of these two things that we do in the distance healing. Well, we can do it either first or second also. The terminology here may lack in describing what this is about, but if you read it through you will come to understand what I am getting at. We create an image of the perfection that is the true being that is the soul, or life-form or spiritual entity or child of God, that has manifested in the physical and lives in/as the client's body. This is to say that you visualize the client as being the perfect being that the heavens would have them be if they had never been touched by anything less than pure ever. If you believe in God, this image of perfection is how God would have made them to enjoy the eternal life that God promises us to enjoy for all of eternity both in physical form and in energy; they may have the halo of a saint like Jesus did and/or the wings of an angel in your image or just be perfectly formed as a human with vitality and perfect health. This image is the only thing that you will think about them as you do the energy work on them. This image is what you will allow your mind to judge them as while you do the quantum healing technique on them from distance or hands-on. This is not the same thing as the tiny image of the client's form that you have in the palm of your hands. This image of perfection is the only thing close to a desired outcome from the treatment that you should ever include in your sessions. Even if the client is the most hideous example of why people should be in prison and how long death can wait to overcome a being, it is in your best interest and the client's best interest to create and hold this image of perfection for them while you are doing the quantum healing work. Even if you think that you know what the specific correction in the specific tissue they need to achieve to get a great result, it is still best to hold this image of perfection for them while you do the quantum healing session on them.

# *Appendix 2*

If you want to create the energy to use for healing to a different place than the hands, it works as well. The hands are a convenient place to achieve the healing energetic as they are easily placed at various positions on a client. If you are holding a baby, it is OK to bring the waves of awareness from your feet to your head to your chest and forearms. This makes sense if the baby is lying across your chest and being braced from rolling down your belly by your forearms as it will bring the healing energetic to the location of the baby more accurately than your hands. Either will work well. If you want to do quantum healing for a dog that is lying across your foot and you are not feeling like a change of your own body position is desirable for your own comfort, you can do the waves backward. I have experimented with doing the waves from the hands to the head and then to the feet and found that I was creating an equivalent energetic at/around my feet that has the same healing-inducing effects. This also lends to the use of self-healing work in quantum healing as you can run the waves of awareness from anywhere (maybe the feet) to any location inside the body that needs some help/healing. When I use to jog a lot late at night, I often jogged on the grassy boulevards in Vancouver. In many places, there are tree roots and other things bringing variations to the plane of the surface beneath the varying lengths of grass. Sometimes I rolled my foot and strained my ankle. If you have ever done this, you may remember the discomfort. I simply used the QH waves of awareness from my feet to my head and then back to my feet while I continued running/limping, and within a block or two, I was always back up to speed with no pain for the rest of my run or signs of strain the next day. It isn't the direction that makes the difference; only the process of consciously feeling/noticing the body in a flowing manner is needed to create the healing energetic. It seems that the further the wave travels and the more fully the physical is felt/noticed, the fuller the energetic becomes. If you concentrate on using the hands-free technique, it may be a good idea to start the waves from the hands at the same time that you start them from the feet and bring them together as one at the crown before arriving at the external location/s to spin the hands-free ball/s. I have done this, and it does work well.

# Appendix 3

When I write or say "physically sighted," I mean to have the ability to see in energy. To be clear, this means that one is able to see with their eyes the variations in the reflections of light that are a result of the subtle energies associated with auras, flowing of energy in the meridians, nonphysical life-forms, and/or any other energetic/psychic/esoteric occurrence or events. I have met many people who have these abilities. Some of them have had them from birth, and others have trained to achieve them. Some have them in some areas, and others have them in other areas. I have met a few people who clearly see and can describe the energies in the auras of others. A few of them had never studied auras or understood what the aura is. One of these people was surprised when I told him that others could not see the auras. Others learned not to talk about what they saw because most people gave them unfriendly feedback such as denial of what they could see, accusations of having made it up, having blurry vision, and being color-blind, being insane, etc. When I say "physically sighted," it is not the same thing as seeing from the mind's eye. Seeing from the mind's eye is totally different in technique but very similar in result. Seeing from the mind's eye, or the third eye, is to get an image of whatever is being viewed inside of your mind. It is a different way of "seeing" in energy that is just as accurate but quite different. "Physically sighted" refers to the data that is received through the eyes onto the retina that is interpreted with the "visible spectrum" (the hues and colors of light rays that are recognized by science as being between ultraviolet and infrared) by some people to different degrees. I have learned how to see energy with my physical vision (with the light that I catch with my eyes) a little bit. Sometimes I can see the shape of energies, and sometimes I can see the color of energies from the information collected on my retinas. But any time I choose to, I can see whatever there is to see, if I know where to look, from my mind's eye.

# Appendix 4

The legs chakra in its internal positions has an effect on our ability to communicate with the physical world in that it is the chakra energy connection to our limbs, which gives us the ability to interact with other physical forms of congealed energies as we choose to. Ya, this sounds a little abstract. The arms and legs chakras have a direct functional relationship with the joints of our limbs. This indirectly allows us to have the mobility to interact with our surroundings physically on an interactive level. The seven internal chakras have a direct functional relationship with our endocrine glands, which indirectly allow us to interact with the physical world metabolically: the seventh chakra with the pineal gland, the sixth with the pituitary gland, the fifth with the thyroid and parathyroid glands (*although I have had some inclination to suspect that the parathyroid may be connected to the internal position of the tenth chakra*), the fourth with the thymus, the third with the pancreas, the second with the gonads, and the first with the adrenals. (*When the chakras are in balance, it will pull the glands toward balanced and correct functioning and secretion of hormones. This can be done several ways. You can try doing it by artificially manipulating the secretions of the glands with various substances to adjust their secretions, thereby simulating the correct balance to attract the correct energy of balance to affect the chakras and thus get them into balance. Another way is to do yoga asanas correctly so that you massage the glands [and the organs that they control] so that proper circulation occurs and the tissue can cleanse itself of built-up waste and toxins so that it can repair itself. This will allow the correct secretions to be possible. When all the influences that direct the functioning of the glands to secrete hormones are in alignment, the energy balance will help to naturally maintain a balance energetic in the chakras. The other way is to balance the chakras first, and the increased vibration of energy will quickly pull the functioning of the glands into alignment. With the chakras active and aligned, the improved secretions of the*

*glands allow a rapid improvement in the physical function and repair of the*
*physical body. That is why it is so much easier to perform your asanas after doing*
*your chakra meditations. But be warned—if you are doing your asanas correctly,*
*the hormonal secretions will produce the effects that the asanas are designed to*
*produce. So please understand both the proper procedure to perform asanas and*
*the effects that are associated with the practices.*) The legs chakra allows us to
move through the world to explore our passions via its alignment with the
individual chakras of our legs, each being located in a physical joint that if
mobile can move us toward physical locations. The utility of this relationship
becomes understood when you explore the concept of following your heart
to reach your heart's desires; people whose hearts have been broken too
many times often fail to move forward in any direction. The metaphor is
often recognized before the actual weakness in the joints, but it occurs at
the same rate. The arms chakra, which is basically located at the base of the
tongue (*the tongue being the orifice of the heart in Taoist and Chinese medicine*
*theory*), is our other first step, next stage, in access to our surroundings in the
strictly physical sense. The energetic connection between our arms chakra
and our arms' chakras is the link that allows us the ability to manipulate our
physical surroundings more succinctly. When we are damaged emotionally
or intellectually so that our desire to subtly manipulate the physicality of
our world is coming from an imbalance in the heart, our physical form
shows it with a loss of functionality of our hands or arms. (*The heart organ*
*is the home of the mind hence an imbalance in the heart will effect the intellect.*
*The heart organ's energetic imbalance will cause an energetic disturbance in the*
*tissue where the arms chakra exists setting it's energy out of harmony and thus*
*interfering with the energies of the arm charkas and their ability to correctly*
*manifest interactions of the arms in relation to the external reality of the physical*
*world. As the positive emotions of the heart are joy honor and sincerity it follows*
*that when one's heart is in balance their arm and hand motions will be gentle*
*steady and firm, while one with a heart imbalance fostering the negative heart*
*emotions of hastiness arrogance and cruelty may well have more awkward and*
*less stable hand and arm movements. It also follows that their experience of*
*interacting with the physical world may be less enjoyable, both for them and for*
*that which they interact with.*) The soul chakras, or the external chakras that
are identified as the 8th, 9th 10th, 11th, and 12th chakras have the task/
ability to connect us to the other aspects of reality than the physical. Each
brings it's own gifts and can be inhibited by various aspects of our pathology.
By clearing and activating them we can help to clear such pathology and
gain conscious access to their gifts of perception and communication.

# Appendix #5

Sequence for practice:

Invite the pure white light to come in through the top, allowing it to fill up your physical body.

Allow red light enter and fill your body from the bottom.

Have the red and the white to merge together forming an effervescent pink glow.

Allow that pink to fill your entire body and expand out to fill up your aura.

As you inhale through your mouth, focus on how your body feels from your feet to the crown of your head and then to your hands several times with each inhale.

Spin the accumulated energetics and pay attention to their presence as you exhale.

Sense the first chakra, accumulate it into a spear and have it spin, intend that it continues to do so.

Sense the second chakra, accumulate it into a spear and have it spin, intend that it continues to do so.

Sense the third chakra, accumulate it into a spear and have it spin, intend that it continues to do so.

Sense the fourth chakra, accumulate it into a spear and have it spin, intend that it continues to do so.

Sense the fifth chakra, accumulate it into a spear and have it spin, intend that it continues to do so.

Sense the sixth chakra, accumulate it into a spear and have it spin, intend that it continues to do so.

Sense the seventh chakra, accumulate it into a spear and have it spin, intend that it continues to do so.

Sense the eighth chakra, accumulate it into a spear and have it spin, intend that it continues to do so.

Sense the ninth chakra, accumulate it into a spear and have it spin, intend that it continues to do so.

Sense the tenth chakra, accumulate it into a spear and have it spin, intend that it continues to do so.

Sense the eleventh chakra, accumulate it into a spear and have it spin, intend that it continues to do so.

Sense the twelfth chakra, accumulate it into a spear and have it spin, intend that it continues to do so.

Sense the leg's chakras, accumulate them into spears and have them spin, intend that they continue to do so.

Sense the arm's chakras, accumulate them into spears and have them spin, intend that they continue to do so.

Move the soul charkas into their internal positions.

Move the minor charkas into their internal positions.

Adjust the chakra's alignment into their most comfortable correct internal positions within the 14/13 chakra position model.

Continue with the multiple spiraling waves of awareness during your inhales through the mouth.

Continue with the spinning of the energy balls as you exhale on each breath.

Place the energy balls where you choose to, or where your intuition tells you to place them.

Remember who you truly are.

# Testimonials

Some words from students of quantum healing level 1 classes and other recent classes taught by the author, Dr. Douglas Perry, DTCM.

I had lower back spasms when I first arrived on the first day. I had a healing on the area and found the pain had diminished somewhat. I had a second healing the next day and was almost pain free. I was amazed at how quickly I was able to learn the material and that it is immediately applicable.

—**Helen F.,** September 2008, level 1

Fun format, always managed to get the class back on track. The long-term effect will be (hopefully) less tingling (pins and needles) in extremities. The sessions did help lessen them overnight, and backache was diminished.

—**Laine,** September 2008, level 1

Now I know who I am and where we have to go one day. It's enlightenment and meeting your true self. It makes your vision, thoughts, and thinking very clear. It makes you a better person. This course tells you that there is always a solution for any problem and any issue that is within you. Douglas M. Perry is a wonderful person, wonderful and very knowledgeable person. His communication skills are very good. Whatever he has learned in so many years, students are fortunate to receive that knowledge in just two and a half days.

—**Savita,** 2008, level 2

It was a good experience and I enjoyed it very much.

—**James Ang,** level 2 audit, 2008

---

Things that I had clung on to without me knowing left and are gone. I also acquired knowledge that is extremely special to me through conformation from Doug Perry's vast knowledge. Doug is an awesome guy and demonstrates vast knowledge and integrity in his teaching.

—**Remy Godin,** level 2, 2008

---

Enhanced energy and quality of sleep. An amazing journey at the heart of truth, love, and light. Behold, be ready and enjoy the trek of a lifetime!

—**Odette Blier,** level 2, 2008

---

My opportunity to release negative energetics and release the stresses on my body felt great. Also, thanks to the instructor's daughter, my ankle feels better. The meditations put me in touch with a level of spirituality that would have been unattainable without Doug's thoughtful direction.

—**Rick Mackowichuk,** level 2 audit, 2008

---

Thank you. To make this connection is indescribable. Everything is different now. Everything. My spirit has been lifted and lifted again and where it lands—nobody knows, thanks. I am so grateful for this knowledge and my own willingness. I know these will be a perfect match. Thank you, Doug. I am so glad to meet you, my honor.

—**Jessica Mckenzie,** level 2, 2008

---

Yes, indeed, I did. Could not sleep—felt too good. Wanted to be awake to enjoy the delicious feeling of happiness in my body.

—**Imogen Whyte,** 2008

---

The pain in my tummy went away the first time I got a healing. My right ear cleared up more than it had. My sore throat ran away. I enjoyed the class very much. You will definitely see me again in other classes. I plan on carrying on and using the techniques daily, as well as helping others with their vibrations.

—**Ashley Reid,** 2008

By the end of the two days, I definitely felt calmer, and it felt as if a lot of stress was removed from my body. Every body part that was worked on in the group healing felt better, i.e., chest and between shoulder blades, elbow, head. It was certainly quite an experience, and I would recommend this course to anyone who wants to learn or know more about energy healing. Doug was very clear and concise and was very easy to understand, a great teacher.

—**Wilma MacMillan,** 2008

I had a clearer understanding of my physical situation, my energy body, and the connections of all the situations I find myself in and the energies surrounding me and my environment. I feel a real inner shift, a perception shift, and a sense of inner peace that helps me to let go of issues. I feel compassion and forgiveness enveloping my being.

—**Regina B. Reuke,** Burnaby, 2008.

It's been three weeks since I participated in the quantum healing level 1 workshop. Although I have always been aware of energy around my hands, I had not previously practiced a specific modality. This workshop served as a wonderful first exposure to the application of specific technique in moving energy for the purpose of healing. I also found the chakra alignment practices very energizing and beneficial, and am still able to feel the energy shifting within me as I do the practices.

Since the workshop, I have noticed that my gallbladder discomfort appears to have subsided. I believe the healing exercises we did gave support and worked well in conjunction with other practices I have been doing, including Kundalini yoga, acupuncture/acupressure massage, and meditation. Although I had already been doing the other practices prior to the workshop, this seems to have provided a turning point. On another note, my dog had a crisis brought on most likely by heat exhaustion about a week ago, and I became afraid I would lose her. I applied the healing techniques as taught by Doug, and by the next afternoon, she was refreshed enough to go for our usual walk in the woods. Given her age, her recovery was considerably more rapid than I would have normally expected. I noticed that she seems particularly receptive to the energy healing, becoming totally relaxed as if blissed-out and licking my hands and face when we have completed the healing. I am very much looking forward to level 2 and a deeper learning of these principles!

—**Kate F.,** Burnaby, June 2008

I noticed strengthening in areas of my body that previously I had difficulties with. I could also feel energy movement in my body where I have difficulties getting it to move. Most noticeably, I had a drastic increase in my ability to feel and see the energetic or subtle world, energy fields, auras. This is definitely an area that I've got to sharpen to help my other energy practices. Just spending the first of two days in class made my visualizations much clearer and my ability to move the energy in my regular practice much smoother than usual. During this practice, the results were much more powerful.

—**Fritz Paesch,** 2007

I felt overall calm. My back and neck feel better. Also, my stomach feels better. It opened to me a new way to see the world. The class was great. The concepts were explained in a very clear manner. The instructor was really careful on every student's particular need and able to answer competently every question.

—**Stefano Zanetti,** Burnaby, 2007

Throughout the seminar, I felt many various types of shifts of energy and freeing of blockages. The experience was undoubtedly healing on many levels. Doug provides a secure vehicle to experience a very challenging and power-packed course. His instruction I found to be very precise and direct. I came away feeling that I had really learned something significant and practically useful on our journey to greater awareness. I found him to be very sincere, a good source of wisdom. Well done, Doug, thank you!

—**Ken Salmon,** July 2007

I did experience relief in the neck and upper back where I had massive pain; the edge was taken off.

—**Elda E. De Paschoal,** July 2007

I have an in-depth sense of coming home into my being fully reclaiming and accepting my power connections with self and source. Doug, you did an excellent job of facilitating and developing an awesome experience. Thank you for all your support. The class was a very gentle and powerfully integrating experience.

—**Kathryn Polischuk,** July 2007

I experienced an increased energy level and focus. Doug is an excellent teacher and facilitator. Thanks!

—**G. Major,** July 2007

Overall charging and realignment of body. Don't have any major health concerns. Worked on specific areas that needed treatment during the class. Great class for being more in tune with body and mind. Great class for spiritual development. Invaluable amount of knowledge presented. Thanks, Doug!

—**Andrea Koreova,** July 2007

A lot of my body aches dissipated. My throat chakra became stronger along with my voice and inner sense of people listening to what I said. My senses of the possible and reality were expanded. I was profoundly awakened to my power to move energy.

—**Michael Paulse,** July 2007

Absolutely, I feel calmer, reconnected; and my body and spirit feel very refreshed. I like feeling that energy in my chakras, and I'm certain that a remarkable healing has taken place in me today. Good classmates as well. I am really an outdoors freak, so it's difficult for me to sit still, and I get bored easily. Doug kept my attention, and the material was very important to learn. Thanks, Doug.

—**Carol Kitchen,** July 2007

After this class, I am feeling a sense of well-being. I have not been well since a dental mishap for over a year. The work is very profound, both physically and spiritually. The best part was developing the knowing that one can heal oneself, and that's my goal.

—**Deborah Fan,** quantum healing workshop participant, Vancouver, May 2006

Very good systematic way to give yourself and others a tune-up; to light up your energy centers for high frequency healing, wow, a lifetime tool for health and awareness. Thank you, Doug.

—**Laurie Pryce,** May 2006

Excellent all round. Thank you. Doug's knowledge of the variety of energy healing systems used by the different cultures in today's world is immense. With this, he is able to put together a professional, informative yet simple-to-understand course. A definite recommendation to all those interested.

—**Jason Gill,** 2006

In a sense of clarity, I feel great. My body feels fully recharged, and the path that I'm on I'm definitely going to continue. I am going to recommend it to all my planetary brothers and sisters. Thanks, Doug!

—**Martina Moravkova,** 2006

My hips leveled, and my shoulders felt more relaxed. I feel centered and happy. It was great. It is exciting how easy it is to do.

—**Valeska Gauthier,** 2006

I felt profound shifts in my awareness of myself and others. I could feel much more energy in my whole body and experienced many insights. Doug has a great depth of knowledge and experience that was great to call upon.

—**Lauren Evanow,** 2005

I experienced levels of high vibration and peaceful stillness.

—**Peter Froese,** quantum healing workshop participant, Vancouver, 2005

I experienced release in tension in my shoulders, neck, and heart area. I experienced a feeling of lightness, peace, and deep relaxation by the last class. I really enjoyed Doug's instruction; he kept everything on track.

—**Rose Ananda,** heart quantum healing workshop participant, Vancouver, 2005

I felt more aligned and less stiffness. I felt more empowered to regain my own health and strength. Thank you, Doug!

>—**Revel Kunz,** quantum healing workshop
>participant, Vancouver 2005

I enjoyed this class. Found some things really difficult, but know I need to practice. I was quite surprised at the amount of energy that we could generate. I enjoyed the instruction from Doug. You are very patient and understanding and made the class enjoyable with a few laughs as well as the serious side. Thanks.

>—**Marjorie Mc Nichol,** quantum healing workshop
>participant, Vernon, May 21-22, 2005

Wonderful workshop. I had never worked with chakras before, but the experience I had with them were powerful and lasting. The power in the energy system of our own body is amazing. I was very surprised and learned a lot. I appreciated your openness to learn new things about the system from your students. The pace was *fast*, very high-level learning curve. I was surprised how quickly it becomes easy to shift one's energy levels. Lots of fun; thanks, Doug, for giving the power to the individual.

>—**Mary-Allana Holmes,** quantum healing workshop
>participant, Vernon, May 21-22, 2005

Through learning the practice of quantum healing, I was able to clear energy that was blocked in my throat and face for many decades. I had learned and practiced many other energetic systems, and in only two days of quantum healing practice, I cleared this longtime blockage.

>—**Lorraine Ballantine, Nelson, BC,** quantum healing
>workshop participant, Vernon, May 21-22, 2005

Similar to Quantum-Touch but with the added techniques and slightly different approach Doug brings, I was able to breakthrough to a much higher level of healing ability.

>—**Rob Barnes, Kelowna, BC,** quantum healing workshop
>participant, Vernon, May 21-22, 2005

Thank you, Doug, for allowing me this opportunity to put more pieces together and to demonstrate so much correction in your method of teaching. Personally, I really was able to appreciate the earth's energy in a more sentient healing modality to our human form than ever before. The content was so full yet layered together so well that learning was a pleasure, not a trial. I would recommend this to anyone.

—**Deb Specht,** quantum healing workshop participant, Vernon, May 21-22, 2005

Great presentation—kept course moving and interesting! Thank you!

—**Rick Malcowichuk**

After almost every area of my body received a treatment, I feel I have more energy and generally feel better.

—**B Lea**

Discomforts in shoulders, neck, and right leg much improved, if not completely gone. Feel peaceful, satisfied, able to see things more clearly in regard to energy around us. Excellence of the first degree. Thank you.

—**Bob Lea**

I feel way more "clarity" and focused in the present. I feel more energized than I have been in the last two months. The energy work done on my jaw nerve subsided the pain. It's great to see that you qualify "what you mean," and "what we think you mean" is indeed on par.

—**Susan Pabuick**

I like helping to teach the level 2 classes, when I was younger my dad made me come and help him with the Quantum Healing seminars. I did it but it really wasn't my thing. After taking level 2 and the teachers training I can appreciate what the work really is and understand that it is important. I was often surprised at how impressed the students in the classes were with what we do in the classes and the healing results that they got. I have been getting energy healing when ever I asked as far back as I can remember, and it works. As a teen I am starting to realize that most people have no idea what the world of energy healing is and I am glad that I have been trained into it.

—**Hannah Perry,** Teachers Training Audit
Edmonton 2008

I would describe Doug as an intuitive teacher who is gently guiding yet focused without being forcefully formatted. Though this is not my preferred method of learning, it is definitely effective. He is also extremely flexible and open to the teaching and learning process during instruction, which enables you to feel like you are growing and contributing to the learning process as opposed to being indoctrinated with a personally filtered version of the modality he is teaching.

—**Jennifer Larson,** Reiki masters class, October 2008

I value Doug's teaching to be true, efficient, and effective. Doug demonstrates a vast knowledge in energy healing and physical, which makes the class very interesting, which also makes him able to guide and answer an extensive amount of questions and be able to relate with all students. I am very thankful for your teaching and your time.

—**Remy Godin,** Reiki masters class, October 2008

# *Results*

Most physical problems respond very quickly to quantum healing. Realigning of bones, swollen tissue, limited motion, pain, and tightness all usually improve during the session and continue to improve after the treatment. Sometimes emotional blocks are released during a session. I have seen TMJ, frozen shoulder, abscessed tooth, Crohn's, headaches, and poor vision drastically improve during and after sessions. I even had a client feel some sensation in a part of her leg after one session that had been numb for years.

The results vary depending on the condition and the overall health of the client. If the clients' overall health and their spirit are both low, they may not hold the results as well as a vibrant, happy person. If a client is feeling guilty or undeserving of healing, they likely won't respond as well or retain the results as long. I have seen good, unbelievable results in clients that I never would have believed were possible, and they never expected. A few times, I have also seen very little results for conditions that I had always gotten great results for on similar conditions with other people. From the people that I have taught, I have heard that results are seen on more than 90 percent of the treatments given.

Sometimes the results from quantum healing take a few days to manifest. I have had clients reluctantly pay for sessions and say that they "didn't feel much and definitely don't feel any better," Two or three days later, they phone me and tell me about the fantastic improvements that increased daily! Sometimes the correction that takes place energetically takes some time to affect the tissue to the extent that it corrects itself enough for the person to notice an improvement.

Information about the writer is available at
*www.dougperry.name, www.ylfes.com, www.quantum-healing.name,* and at
*www.arborfieldlight.com.*

E-mail contact: *dougperry_dtcm@yahoo.com*
Phone contact: 604-568-2525

CPSIA information can be obtained at www.ICGtesting.com
Printed in the USA
LVOW071807200911

247103LV00005B/132/P